Cancer Diagnosis
and
Memories of a
Pathologist

By

Peter Yellinek

Copyright © 2024 *Peter Yellinek*
All Rights Reserved.

This book is subject to the condition that no part of this book is to be reproduced, transmitted in any form or means; electronic or mechanical, stored in a retrieval system, photocopied, recorded, scanned, or otherwise. Any of these actions require the proper written permission of the author.

All personal names in the following narrative are fictitious.

To my wife,

who supported me through all my labors.

To our children, to know a little more about my work, and for our grandchildren, to move forward with courage.

Contents

Introduction 5
Chapter 1: The Road to Becoming a Pathologist 6
Chapter 2: Residency Training 12
Chapter 3: Assistant Pathologist 24
Chapter 4: The Draft Board 35
Chapter 5: Harry 43
Chapter 6: The Union 57
Chapter 7: Moonlighting 65
Chapter 8: Teaching and Research 83
Chapter 9: My Immediate Boss 100
Chapter 10: The Joys of a Director of Pathology and Laboratory   114
Chapter 11: Oncology 136
Chapter 12: Other Events and Observations 146
Chapter 13: The Job Search 169
Chapter 14: Hospital Administrators 188
Chapter 15: "The Second Time is Easy" 193
Chapter 16: Lab Inspection and Sundry Tidbits 214
Chapter 17: The Business and Medicine 231
Chapter 18: Some Trends in Pathology 240
Conclusion 251
A Personal Note 255

Introduction

Pathologists make the diagnosis on tissues removed from patients in surgery, they control laboratory tests of blood and other fluids, and they perform autopsies. Some pathologists act as coroners or medical examiners in support of the law, or they do research and teach at medical schools, or they serve as consultants in pharmaceutical or other industries.

This memoir tells the stories taken from the life of an MD pathologist in the span of 42 years of practice in hospitals and academic centers, including episodes from 25 years of acting as Director of a Department of Pathology and Laboratories, with special attention to cancer diagnosis and therapy. Some stories cover the events associated with training the residents in pathology; others speak of the mysteries of basic science research and occasional aberrations in scientific publications. The memoir also touches upon interesting social encounters, displaying the attitudes in a segment of our society. In addition, there are personal observations with comments about the great changes in medical practice over the past fifty years, changes which transformed medicine into "healthcare" and introduced the concept of "managed care", where the physician has become an employe who may be allotted only a short, limited time for a patient visit.

Chapter 1

The Road to Becoming a Pathologist

Long before one thinks of becoming a pathologist, there must be a desire to follow the path into higher education and choose to study medicine and become a physician. There are many reasons why young people decide to pursue a medical career, but I can only speak of my own motivation.

My awareness and first memories of a 'doctor' came in early childhood, when a series of minor ailments, either simple colds with fever and headache or a painful earache, that compelled my parents to take me to a physician's office. The doctor would order that I stay in bed and receive a medicine, which I recall as some white powder that was mixed with water. The bitter-tasting medicine, like a miracle in a story, brought down the fever; my headache would vanish, and soon, I would be able to jump out of bed and once again feel like my usual self. I believed that the doctor's bitter powder had a 'magic power,' somewhat like the magic in the fables that my mother used to read to me before bedtime.

Not all my childhood encounters with the doctors were agreeable, though. I had two surgical procedures that were so frightful, that I could still remember how the first one happened when I was about five years old, following an accident. I had a habit of happily running through the length of our apartment and stopping myself with both arms extended against the glass of our kitchen door. As I got bigger, my habit of leaning into the glass door led to an accident where my right arm smashed through the glass. When I hastily pulled my arm back, blood began to stream from my wrist, and the sight of it filled me with a terrible fright and a wave of nausea. My mother, hearing the crash of broken glass and my wailing, ran quickly after me. She carried me into the bathroom, fetched from the medicine cabinet a bandage, and wound it tightly around the bleeding wrist. A taxi was called, and I was taken to the doctor's office. The doctor tied a rubber band around my arm, unwound the bloody bandage, and spread some white powder all over the wound. Then he started touching and poking with tweezers all under the broken skin, and strangely, I felt no pain. The wound was numb, like a piece of wood. Again, I thought that the doctor's white powder had some sort of magic in it. While my mother held me on her lap, the doctor placed my arm on a table covered with clean white sheets and started picking out of the wound tiny splinters of glass.

This awful search went on for some time, till he could find no more glass. Then the doctor made a few stitches with a needle and thread inside the wound and placed several small metal clamps to hold together the skin. He bandaged the wrist and put the arm into a sling that hung over my shoulder. My arm remained in the sling for many days, till I was again taken to the doctor's office, and he removed the bandage and skin clamps. A jagged, one-inch-long scar with clamp marks still marks the inner side of my right wrist.

My second experience with surgery was no less distressing. I was ten years old when it was decided that my constantly swollen tonsils and adenoids had to be taken out. The operation took place in a surgeon's private office. My whole body and arms were wrapped around with a white sheet, and, like a mummy, I was placed to sit on the lap of a male nurse, who held me snugly by holding his arms around my body. Then, the doctor suddenly came from behind and covered my entire face with a large white mask made of wire and gauze. Inside the mask was a frightening darkness, and worse, there was a horrible acrid smell, a smell that made me choke and retch. I heard the doctor say loudly:

"Now breathe in deeply, and count to twenty! Count loud, so I can hear you!"

The mask was held tight against my face, and I had no choice but to obey. I started counting, and I don't know how far I went… When I woke up, I felt dizzy, and when I was freed from the white sheet and put on my feet, I saw the whole room turn around me. I could not stand or walk without being supported. We went home by taxi, and every time the car made a turn, I felt nauseous. Our apartment was on the third floor, and when the elevator abruptly stopped, I felt my whole stomach come up into my throat. I spit out and made a puddle of dark, nearly black blood on the floor. I was cleaned up and put to bed and slept for a few hours. I woke up with a sore throat and was soon offered some ice cream, which felt very soothing.

By the age of ten, I was fully aware that my doctor's medications carried no magic at all. This was reinforced after I read my favorite novel, Karl May's *"Winnetou,"* in which a shaman had an amulet that was supposed to have 'magic powers,' but it was clear that the magic existed only in the story. By the time I was about twelve, I had learned some real facts about doctors and the medical profession. Physicians were well respected and very much in demand in every part of the world. It was this last insight that would induce me to think about becoming a medical doctor. That profession made a perfect fit with my desire to leave the place where I was born and go to live in a better world. I always remember how my parents frequently talked about wanting to go to "America," which, for some to me unknown reason was not possible. I also could not forget the horrors brought upon most of my family during the Second World War. My parents were taken away, and only after the war ended and they did not return, I found that they were brutally murdered. Then I became aware that I was lucky to survive, only through kindness and decency of a few brave and exceptional people.

During the last few years of high school, I began to recognize my affinity for the study of sciences. Physics, chemistry, and biology were my favorites. When the question came up, what course would I choose at the university, I had no doubt or hesitation. I was determined to study medicine and become a doctor. With that in mind, I took good care of my grades, to qualify for acceptance into the medical school. While in medical school, I never thought of choosing a specialty. One could begin to think of a specialty only after graduation, following the experience of a year of internship in a hospital.

My first engagement in the practice of medicine came during the customary "rotating internship," a one-year rotation through various specialties, including internal medicine, general surgery, obstetrics and gynecology, pediatrics and the emergency room in a hospital. During that year, there was lots of contact with patients, many sleepless nights, and many overtime hours spent entering patients' histories and physicals into hospital charts, all by longhand. The remaining time was spent reading medical journals and textbooks in the hospital library to expand medical knowledge.

With all that activity, I soon realized that teaching, working in a laboratory, and continuing to learn and do some research would be a most pleasing way to put to practice my medical knowledge. A survey of all medical specialties revealed that pathology offered a career most suitable to what I liked to do. Working with a microscope and making a diagnosis felt like interesting and challenging work. Practicing pathology in a hospital affiliated with a medical school would offer the opportunity to teach, do research, and work in a medical laboratory. It was the attraction to all these activities that affirmed my decision to seek a residency training in pathology. There was yet another advantage: pathology offered the possibility of having an academic career, and furthermore, medical schools were often located in larger urban centers, with access to cultural events which I liked.

Looking deeper into the specialty of pathology, I could see that it was a very broad field, encompassing all specialties of medicine. Pathologists receive samples of tumors or diseased tissue for diagnosis not only from general surgeons, but also from specialists for ear, nose and throat, gynecologists, eye doctors, neurologists, dermatologists, urologists, orthopedists, pulmonary specialists, and even cardiologists. In pathology, one would have the opportunity to use, maintain and enlarge all the knowledge acquired in medical school. Thus, I decided to apply for a residency in pathology in a hospital affiliated with a medical school, so that already during training, there would be an opportunity to teach and do research.

The above-described career path towards choosing a specialty in medicine was typical and customary in the sixties of the twentieth century. In the last fifty years, a rotating internship has become a thing of the past. It used to be in the sixties that a young MD coming out of a rotating internship could immediately open an office of 'general practice' and begin to see patients. Nowadays, the 'general practice' of many years ago has become a specialty called "Family Practice," and it requires residency training, just like 'Emergency Medicine,' surgery, psychiatry, etc. Now, every physician becomes a specialist. Currently, the pathway leading to a medical specialty has undergone a great change. Already during the senior year of medical school, well before getting an MD degree, the medical student has to decide and choose a specialty before having had any experience in the practice of medicine.

The student applies for specialty training at multiple places, and the participating hospitals offer a "matching program" whereby the students are informed of their placement location. Sometimes a student's choice of specialty turns out to be quite different from what she or he expected while still in medical school. Many would have made a better choice if they had been given a year of rotating internship.

Chapter 2

Residency Training

In 1963, I was accepted into a residency training program in anatomic and clinical pathology in New York City, at a hospital affiliated with a medical school. There were six novice residents, and the total number of residents in the entire four-year program was more than twenty. Half the residents were American-born, and the other half were immigrants from various countries.

On the first day, all novices were met by the Chief Resident, and he introduced us to the professors and other senior residents. He also gave us the schedule and various instructions, including the rules of the department. In the first year, a resident learns to perform autopsies; in the second year, one learns to make diagnoses of surgically removed tissue and cell smears (cytology); and in the third and fourth years, one acquires the skills in the clinical laboratory testing and management, while continuing to study and improve on diagnostic skills in surgical pathology, cytology and autopsies.

My boss during the first year was Dr. Bernhard Grabner, a middle-aged Associate Professor in charge of autopsy training. He was a tall, slim, man, neatly dressed, with a bowtie, and he spoke with a British accent. He was very friendly, and a few days after I met him, he offered me to do research in his department and explained that I would participate in the electron microscopic study of amyloid. The object was to search for the origin and structure of amyloid, a mysterious substance that invades many organs and causes death by destroying a large part of the heart or liver or kidneys. At that time, there was no laboratory test for amyloid, and the diagnosis could be made either by organ biopsy or at autopsy. Amyloid accumulation in the brain was suspected to be the cause of Alzheimer's disease, and still now, more than 60 years later, we have the same suspicion, without a definite proof. A full understanding of the cause of Alzheimer's disease awaits further research.

Research had to be done after regular work hours, and the Chairman of the Department of Pathology offered a small supplemental stipend for those of us who were willing to volunteer. The residents' salaries at the time were about 3,500 dollars in the first year of training. For comparison, an office clerk/typist was at that time earning about 4,000 dollars per year. Many residents who were married and had children, instead of volunteering in research, preferred to earn extra money by "moonlighting," that is, making evening house calls as general practitioners, or serving as 'house physicians' during night shifts in small private hospitals that had no residency training programs.

I admitted to Dr. Grabner that, while I was very familiar with the regular light microscope, the electron microscope was an instrument that I had never seen before. Dr. Grabner assured me that it was not a problem. He would assign a mentor to instruct me on how to use the instrument, and he introduced me to a young Assistant Professor, Dr. Yoshi Komura, who was doing research in his department. Within the next two months, Dr. Komura taught me all there was to know about the electron microscope, including the special method of tissue preparation.

Even before showing me the instrument, Dr. Komura warned me that the electron microscope used high voltage (200,000 volts) and not to be frightened by a deafening thunder-like noise that would occasionally resound from it due to high voltage discharge into the ground. He said, not to worry, the instrument was securely grounded. The thunderous machine was nine feet tall, and with its high voltage cable, vacuum pump and chamber, built-in camera, and a console table, it occupied a specially designed darkroom with steel reinforced floor. The instrument had such enormous magnifying power, that it could reveal objects as small as 0.1 nanometer (one ten-millionth of a millimeter). The magnified images were created by electrons streaming from the tip of a Tungsten filament into the vacuum chamber, and then passing through an ultra-thin section of the examined tissue sample. The image was viewed on a fluorescent screen, very much like in an X-ray viewing chamber, and areas of interest were photographed and captured with black and white film. Teaching me about tissue preparation for electron microscopy, Dr. Komura warned that I better have a keen eye and a steady hand, and above all, lots of patience while trying to cut and handle the fragile ultra-thin tissue sections. *

The tissue for my research was obtained at an autopsy of a patient who died of massive amyloid accumulation in his liver. Under a regular light microscope, the amyloid could be recognized by its amorphous

---

* The preparation of the tissue for electron microscopy was a long process, a whole adventure. It required that a small tissue sample of about 2 mm be set into a mold with epoxy resin that would, after several days, harden into cement. The cement with the embedded tissue is then cut by a special microtome, using diamond knives, to produce extremely thin sections, which would be floated onto the water in a tiny trough. Since diamond knives were expensive, being a novice, I had to learn to produce cheap disposable knives made of thick glass that became unusable after only 5 or 6 sections of epoxy cement. Thus, in the process of learning electron microscopy, I became an expert glass cutter. The tissue sections were floated on water, and had to be of purple or silver color, just like the very fine film of oil that is often seen floating on filthy water in a harbor. The purple or silver color was a sign that the section was thin enough to allow the passage of electrons in the microscope. A section had to be delicately picked up from the surface of the water with a small carbon-coated copper grid that fit into the chamber of the electron microscope. This entire procedure required several weeks to master.

appearance and a few staining properties that it shared with various other biological substances in nature. Electron microscopy could perhaps offer a clue to the nature of amyloid by exposing the fine details of its structure. Dr. Grabner showed me some ill-defined electron images of amyloid that he obtained, displaying the form of thin filaments. A few other American researchers also found that amyloid was composed of fine filaments. The problem was that the researchers in France had published images of amyloid, showing only tiny round, donut-shaped rings and no filaments at all. The question was: which one of these tiny structures represented amyloid? Over the next several months, I made different preparations of amyloid by homogenizing it in a refrigerated ultracentrifuge. By changing the speed of the centrifuge, I was hoping to find the ring forms described in France. The research was a slow and tedious process, but I plunged into it with excitement and determination. In the lab, I kept a notebook where I recorded each procedure and documented the findings by electron photographs. My preparations began to show sharp, thin filaments, but there was no trace of ring forms.

One day, a resident colleague told me that my boss, Dr. Grabner, was seen reading my research notebook and taking notes from it. I thought that it was his prerogative. Several months later, I was told by a senior resident that Dr. Grabner had attended a conference on amyloid in Europe, had apparently presented some results of his work, and that his presentation would be published. The galley proofs of the publication had been returned to our department for corrections, and I went to look at them. To my surprise, I found that all the pictures to be published were those I had recently obtained, and Dr. Grabner was listed as the sole author. I spoke to my mentor, Dr. Komura, and he suggested that I inquire about the authorship rules at the office of "The Chief", the informal name we used for the Chairman of the Department.

The Chief had an immediate solution: since the images and corresponding text came from my work, and since Dr. Komura was my research instructor, the final publication should include both of our names as co-authors. It was customary that Dr. Grabner, who presented the work at the conference, should be listed as the first author. The Chief said that he would talk to Dr. Grabner and straighten out the authorship.

My first impression of research habits in an academic institution was somewhat disturbing, but I learned from it that the sole authorship was highly coveted, because most research was done by a team of several people. From then on, as part of my apprenticeship in research, I purchased a little attaché case, and every night I carried my notebook and all pictures home. I continued the research, hoping that someday I would succeed in finding the ring forms of amyloid and get some new data worthy of publishing.

In my second year of residency, I was assigned to train in diagnostic surgical pathology, together with five other residents. The department was headed by Dr. Josef Moholy, and his associate was Dr. Ian Romer, an experienced senior pathologist. Every morning, all six of us residents would sit around a large table, pass around microscopic slides and discuss our diagnoses. Then, there would be a formal "sign-out conference," where each resident would present his diagnosis for approval and discussion by either Dr. Moholy or Dr. Romer. The final diagnoses would be dictated, typed by a secretary, and signed by the attending pathologist.

In my first week in surgical pathology, there was an incident that had an unexpected outcome. During the morning sign-out conference, Dr. Moholy was called away to receive a visitor in his private office, and while the six of us residents were waiting for him to return, I took one of my cases to the office of Dr. Romer and asked him to help me with the diagnosis. When Dr. Moholy returned to the sign-out conference, I presented the diagnosis, but to my surprise, Dr. Moholy disagreed, and made a different one. I was troubled: it was a tumor of skin, and the difference in diagnosis was important. I had to decide what to do. It was hard to say it, but I admitted that I had asked Dr. Romer for help with the diagnosis. As expected, that struck a raw nerve. Dr. Moholy, right in front of the other five residents, gave me a sharp lecture on how I should never show my assigned cases to any pathologist other than the one doing the sign-out conference. I was completely embarrassed, and I immediately apologized. Dr. Moholy meanwhile kept looking at that same case a little longer, and then quietly changed the diagnosis, accepting the one of Dr. Romer. Later, I felt quite aggrieved, because I did what was right for the patient. It was a very inauspicious beginning of a year of training in diagnostic surgical pathology.

The next day, "The Chief" walked in during the morning sign-out conference, and as was his habit, he greeted us with:

"Everything alright, guys?"

"Well, I have a question…" I said, "I was told, that we should not show our assigned cases to anyone other than the attending pathologist, who does the daily sign-out. Is that a rule?"

"Oh, no!" said The Chief, "You may consult with as many pathologists in our department as you wish! That's how you learn!"

Dr. Moholy promptly cut in:

"Dr. Yellinek was disruptive! He left the room during the sign-out conference and showed a case to Dr. Romer!"

I was taken aback, but quickly gathered my wits:

"Chief, please: Dr. Moholy was called out during the sign-out to meet a visitor in his office. I showed the case to Dr. Romer during the time we waited for Dr. Moholy to return."

There was a stony silence. Dr. Moholy's face turned red. The Chief looked for a moment at Dr. Moholy, and then told him quietly:

"Josef, come with me! In your office!"

They shut the door of the private office and remained there for some time. The six of us residents sat in the conference room and quietly looked at our cases. A few minutes later, Dr. Romer showed up and finished the sign-out conference for that day. That evening, I went home quite upset.

The next morning, as soon as I came in to work, a message was waiting for me, to immediately come to the Chief's office. That meant going from the hospital to the medical school building, about a quarter mile across the campus. Those ten minutes that I had to walk, I was scared. I felt I should never have spoken to the Chief about the whole incident. As soon as I came in and greeted the Chief's secretary, she directed me to see the Chief's main assistant. He asked me to sit down and immediately addressed the issue that sat with a heavy load on my mind:

"Well, you know, for the moment, we thought…" and he spoke slowly and deliberately: "… it would be best for you to continue your surgical pathology training at another institution…" I froze! It flashed through my mind that I was being sacked, thrown out of the residency program. The Chief's assistant continued:

"We have arranged that you train in surgical pathology as a guest resident. Your salary will come from us, but you will be going to Columbia University."

It took me a moment or two to wake up from the shock, and then slowly, it began to sink in... I began to understand that I was to train at an institution that had one of the best surgical pathology departments in the country, a place where every future pathologist could only dream of training.

The Chief's assistant advised me to gather all my belongings and drive the very same morning across town and present myself to Dr. Lattes, the Chairman of the Department of Surgical Pathology at Columbia Presbyterian Hospital. It took almost an hour before I arrived and found parking. By the time I reached the Department of Surgical Pathology, I was again perfectly calm and composed. Dr. Lattes welcomed me and immediately introduced me to his assistant, who then introduced me to other attending pathologists and a large group of residents. The Chief Resident assigned me to a desk with a microscope and handed me the schedule with the rules of the department. As I settled down in my new place, it slowly became clear to me that I was going to train in a department that had a six times larger volume of cases to learn from, than where I started only a few days earlier. I was aware that Dr. Raffaele Lattes, the Chairman of Surgical Pathology at Columbia University, was a world-renowned scholar and expert who published many articles and co-authored a book on the diagnosis of connective tissue tumors.

During that year at Columbia University Hospital, I saw a large number of difficult diagnostic problems and had the opportunity to properly learn how to make a pathologic diagnosis. When that year ended, I returned to my original residency program to continue the final two years of training in clinical laboratory. However, during those last two years of residency, I was allowed to continue visiting Columbia University Hospital every Saturday. There, I would spend the whole day in the Surgical Pathology department, gaining more knowledge and experience by studying the great variety of rare and unusual cases that were regularly set aside for residents' training. It was the studying at Columbia that would eventually give me the confidence to function as a well-qualified diagnostic pathologist and head of a department of pathology.

In the last two years of residency, learning about the clinical laboratory and its various equipment, methodology, and management presented a vast field that was very different from diagnostic surgical pathology. The laboratory had various sections: hematology, chemistry, microbiology, serology, and the blood bank, each with completely different equipment and methods of testing. The blood bank performed compatibility testing between patients and blood donor units and kept tabs on the expiration dates of transfusion products. Chemistry had the largest variety of lab tests and equipment. The microbiology section had to identify bacteria by growth on various nutrients, and serology had an assortment of tests for viruses or serum antibodies. The hematology section had automated counters for red and white blood cells and platelets, and it dealt with blood coagulation testing.

Looking at my fellow residents, I noticed that at Columbia University, all were American born except the Chairman of Surgical Pathology, Dr. Lattes, who was an immigrant and spoke with a sweet Italian accent. At the medical school where I started and then continued my residency training, half of the residents were American-born, and the rest came from abroad, four from China, two from Korea, and one each from Greece, Italy, Japan, Turkey and Yugoslavia. We had only two female residents: one from Greece and one from Nebraska. The latter drove around in a sports Mercedes. How times have changed! Most recent statistics show that 52 percent of pathologists are female, and as of 2019, more than 50 percent of medical students were female.

The residents lived like a large, friendly family. We all hated the food in the hospital cafeteria, and frequently, the whole large group would go out for lunch to a local place that had good pizza or seafood. One of the Chinese residents introduced us to Chinese restaurants, and he taught us to say a greeting and a few basic phrases in Chinese. Our departmental Christmas party was usually catered by an Italian deli, and the two Jewish residents knowingly enjoyed the shrimp, prosciutto, and salami. One Chinese fellow, who was a Jehovah's Witness, happily ate the Italian blood sausage, completely unaware of what it contained. When he asked me what the name of that delicious dark sausage was and where could he buy it, I haltingly answered that I did not know.

The technical staff in the laboratory and the clerical staff in the pathology offices came from all parts of the world. There were two immigrants from the UK. One of them was the lab manager, a middle-aged, highly competent and knowledgeable technologist. She was a tall and well built, good-natured lady, always wearing a smile and willing to teach. She spoke with a stubborn British accent despite having been in the US for more than 15 years. The other British immigrant worked in the pool of secretaries who typed all our pathology reports. A small and slender young woman, blond with a pale face, she not only spoke with a hard British accent, but she took it upon herself to correct (very rightfully) the broken English spoken and written by some of us immigrants.

Fortuitously, I would meet the same secretary about twelve years later, while attending a pathology conference with lectures and courses in San Francisco. Those conferences were usually attended by several graduates from our residency training program, and we always organized an evening out to meet over dinner and get current on our progress. On that occasion, one of our Korean colleagues, Jay, was the last one to arrive for dinner, and since he lived in a nearby suburb, he brought along his wife. He had obvious fun, seeing the surprise on all our faces when we realized that his wife was none other than our former office secretary, Jenny. Jay and Jenny managed to keep their relationship completely secret during all four years of residency training. What I also learned at that dinner was that, way back then, during residency, everyone on the staff called me by the nickname "Hobbit." Jenny hinted that it was the other British lady, the lab manager, who made it up.

In my last four months of residency, I was promoted to the rank of Chief Resident. In that position, I was assigned a newly introduced duty for the Chief Resident: to conduct surgical pathology sign-out conference one day a week with junior residents. This would help me to prepare for work in my next role as an attending pathologist. I anticipated that new duty with great trepidation, for I had to first meet the department head, Dr. Moholy, whom I have not seen ever since the incident that propelled me to Columbia University. Just moments before meeting him, I was relieved as I saw him approaching with a broad smile. He welcomed me with a friendly pat on the shoulder and loudly announced:

"Good to have you with us, Peter! We can really use some help!"

"I am glad to be back! Columbia was tough!", and I bit my tongue. Dr. Moholy, however, just kept smiling and behaved as if nothing ever happened between us. The other senior pathologist, Dr. Romer, was kind and pleasant and treated me as an old friend.

Towards the end of the fourth year of residency, the time had come to look for my first job as an attending pathologist. I had several interviews for that position, and as there was at the time a relative shortage of young pathologists in NYC, I was able to get a suitable position in a hospital of my choice. The hospital had a new electron microscope suite with a fully equipped research lab, financed by a wealthy donor, so that I could continue with my research. The hospital was also affiliated with a medical school where I could attend conferences and lectures. My future boss promised to get me an academic appointment at the medical school, with the possibility of actively participating in student teaching.

Chapter 3

Assistant Pathologist

1967 was a significant year for our family. All in sequence, our first child, a beautiful little daughter, was born. I had completed residency training and started my first job as an attending pathologist, and in December of that year, after five long years, Miriam and I had received American citizenship.

My first job as an Attending Pathologist was at a general hospital that also specialized in orthopedic surgery. On the first day of work, my boss, Dr. Donald Dickerman, a soft-spoken, middle-aged man, reaffirmed his promise to get me an academic appointment on the staff of the affiliated medical school where he was a Clinical Associate Professor. My major job was to provide diagnoses in surgical pathology, and I had to supervise and solve problems in the clinical laboratory. The volume of work was not too heavy, and I had enough time to prepare for the specialty board examination in anatomic and clinical pathology.

Nearly one-half of all diagnostic pathology in that hospital involved tissues from orthopedic surgery, particularly tumors of bone, cartilage and connective tissue, and I had the opportunity to enhance my knowledge in that difficult subspecialty. In the clinical laboratory, I met and collaborated with a PhD bacteriologist, who discovered and named two new strains of bacteria that had never been recognized before. He needed help in defining the fine morphologic features of the newly discovered organisms, and I was able to demonstrate them by electron microscopy. Within two years, we jointly published two papers in the Journal of Clinical Bacteriology.

On many evenings, after my regular working hours, I put in some time in the electron microscopy suite and continued my research on amyloid. During that, I had an unusual new experience. One late afternoon, as I walked into the electron microscopy suite, I saw two men who were just about finished with the cleanup of the room. They stood near the door, keenly looking around, obviously making a final check that everything was in good order. Not wanting to interrupt them, I asked if they needed some more time to complete their job. One of them looked at me and said:

"Aah…, no, no, we are done!" and they turned around, carried out the trash bags and left. Before entering the electron microscope enclosure, I noticed that the light microscope was not in its usual place. *Where the hell did they move it?* I thought to myself. When I could not see it on any bench, I ran to the window just in time to see the two men with garbage bags briskly crossing the street below. Well, this operation was done in broad daylight and in a smooth, agreeable, and cool manner. It was just a plain little robbery, not at all frightening, because, luckily, I did not realize what was happening, until it was too late.

I called the hospital security and started surveying the whole room: a small precision scale and a few other little instruments were also missing. Two security men came up, and they praised me for having been so "cool and wise" as not to try to confront the robbers. The security men were very professional: they said that such things were quite common, and anyway, it would be dangerous to try to stop the robbers. I thanked them for their help and good advice. The missing equipment was soon replaced, and the old entry door got a new, better lock.

In the Spring of 1968, I flew to Houston, TX, to take the examination by The American Board of Pathology. The exam took three days, and each evening I joined several friends from New York for a walk around Houston. Walking along, we noticed that in some of the bars, there was a prominent sign in the window: "NO COLORED ADMITTED." After seeing the third such sign, one of my friends from NYC quietly said:

"It feels like I am in a foreign country!"

We continued walking in silence, everyone with their own thoughts. I thought of how lucky I was to have settled in the State of New York… Then I turned my thoughts towards the next day, the final day of the exam. Three weeks later, I received a letter informing me that I was board-certified in Anatomic and Clinical Pathology.*

At that time, the routine workload in surgical pathology had significantly increased, and Dr. Dickerman hired a second Attending Pathologist. It was a lady who had moved to NYC from Ohio, where she and her husband, a surgeon, had practiced for several years in a small rural hospital. They had two pre-teen children, and I could not

---

* Diploma in Anatomic Pathology certifies that a physician is qualified to make pathologic diagnoses on all patients' tissues, body fluids, and cell smears and to perform autopsies. The NY State law (at the time) required that all tissues surgically or otherwise removed from patients must be examined by a certified pathologist and that a diagnostic report be provided to the ordering physician, with a copy placed into the patient's hospital record.

A diploma in Clinical Pathology certifies that a physician is qualified to direct medical laboratories performing all regular tests on patients' blood, urine, and other liquid or solid materials. That includes tests in hematology, chemistry, bacteriology, serology, and blood transfusion compatibility. By law, the test results, expressed in quantitative and qualitative measures, must be provided to the ordering physician with a copy put onto the patient's hospital record.

During the past forty years, the laws concerning medical laboratories have been significantly modified. Senior technologists and PhDs are allowed to become directors of medical laboratories. Pathologists are still required for the diagnosis of tissue or cytology.

understand why a family of two physicians with school-age children would move from a quiet town with fresh air into a crowded city, where the air was filled with black smoke daily spewing from thousands of garbage-burning incinerators. And besides, a physician's income in rural Ohio was more than double of that in NYC. Now, they lived in a small apartment in the East Bronx, where the surgeon got a job in a City Hospital around the corner from their home. My new partner at work was diligent, pleasant and easygoing, and one day, over lunch, she quietly told me why they moved away from Ohio.

Both she and her husband immigrated to the US from Iran and finished their internship and residency training in NYC. Soon thereafter, both found full-time positions in a rural hospital in Ohio. There, they enjoyed the clean air, the low cost of living, and the fact that they could immediately afford a house with a large backyard. Their two children attended a local public school. Both were well-appreciated at work, and their neighbors were polite and always greeted them in a friendly manner. However, over several years, the couple made no headway in social life, and they did not find any local friends. Their two children did well in school, and they played with their schoolmates outside of the house. However, when the children had a birthday party and invited their playmates, the parents of the playmates would politely call and excuse their children for not being able to come. The Iranian couple was never invited into the homes of their neighbors or local co-workers. The boss of the pathologist invited them once for dinner at a restaurant, and the boss of the surgeon invited them once for dinner at his golf club. When the Iranian couple invited their co-workers or neighbors to visit them at home, they would come, but only for a brief stop, barely enough to have a cup of coffee. Finally, my partner told me, she and her husband felt that their family was never accepted as a part of the local community. Perhaps it was, my partner said, because of their different religion -

they were Bahai. Having the feeling of being forever treated as outsiders, they preferred to move back to NYC, which, with its great diversity, made them feel more at home.

By then, I have also learned that an immigrant should not be surprised by an occasional odd or unpleasant incident. In 1963, during our first vacation in the US, Miriam and I experienced one such event. We bought our first car and decided to travel from NYC through Pennsylvania to visit and stay with a friend in Columbus, Ohio. About halfway through the trip, we decided to make an overnight stop in Bedford Springs, PA. Seeing ahead of us a fork in the road, I pulled the car well onto the side, a yard away from the pavement, and stopped to look at the map and see which way to go. A few moments later, I heard a loud, gruff voice coming through the open car window:

"Move on!"

I looked up and saw a policeman with a wide-brimmed hat motioning me to move forward.

"Excuse me! Officer, I just want to…" but he interrupted:

"Move on! MOVE ON!" he yelled with an angry voice. I was stunned, and with the map in my lap, I still hesitated for a moment. Then I saw him slowly pulling his gun out of the holster and lifting it up toward me. Staring at me madly, he screamed:

"NOW!"

I let the map slide onto the floor, grabbed the steering wheel, and took off as fast as I could. I took the right side of the fork: it was closer. Making sure that the policeman did not follow us, Miriam and I slowly recovered from the shock and began to talk. We debated why the policeman (or was it a sheriff?) was so belligerent. We concluded that there was probably more than one reason for his behavior. First, our car had a "foreign" license plate of someone from NYC. Next, the policeman may not have liked the appearance of the driver, which was somewhat unexpected in the rural part of Pennsylvania: a man with curly black hair and dark brown, well-tanned skin, speaking with a foreign accent. It seemed, the policeman was raised and educated to be suspicious of any person who appeared so "different".

After having been in the US for nearly one year, it was our very first time experiencing a person who was so openly hostile, rude, and belligerent. This was a little hard to digest, but we were on vacation and decided not to dwell on it. Within half an hour, we arrived in Bedford Springs and saw that several houses had a "ROOM FOR RENT" sign on the front lawn. Rather than staying in an impersonal motel, we rented a room in a private home, stayed overnight and had breakfast with the family. As we talked with them, we had the impression of very friendly people. We noticed that my appearance and our foreign accent did not seem to bother them at all. Well, we were the guests in a little rural resort.

Speaking of attitudes in the rural US, whether in the Midwest or in the South, or indeed, in any part of the country, one must be prepared for all sorts of experiences. Here is a story that occurred much later, in the mid-eighties, and it did not happen to us but to a couple of our American friends, both born and raised in New Jersey. At the time, we lived in a rural area not far from the Canadian border, and the house next door to ours had changed owners. Soon, we became very friendly with our new neighbors, a young couple with two small preschool children. Our neighbor worked for the IBM corporation, and he was just transferred into the area. He told us that it was customary at IBM to promote and transfer employees about every two years. The acronym IBM, our neighbor explained jokingly, stood for "I've-Been-Moved". Of course, it was not pleasant for the wives and the children of the employees to move and change schools every couple of years, but every good job may have a little downside. A day came when our friendly neighbor was again promoted and transferred, this time to Alabama. We liked each other and continued to stay in touch both by correspondence and occasionally by phone. What they reported during their two years in Alabama was quite shocking. They made no friends and had no close social contact with any of their local neighbors or co-workers. The boss at IBM invited them once for dinner, not at his house, but at his club. No local family ever invited them into their house except a few co-workers who had come from the North. Briefly, they were "Yanks" and felt treated "worse than strangers". Of course, they could not wait for the next IBM transfer. Finally, they were transferred to Connecticut, where they resumed a normal social life.

By the end of 1968, I was still waiting for the academic appointment at the medical school, which Dr. Dickerman promised when I accepted the job. Along with my regular work, I was able to attend evening lectures and conferences at the school, but I felt that a formal appointment would be important for my future career. A couple of times, when I approached Dr. Dickerman and asked about it, he assured me that it was imminent, "it should be coming now, any time", he said, and he "just recently spoke" about my appointment with the Chairman of the Department.

In the Spring of 1969, after attending an evening lecture at the medical school, I garnered enough courage to approach the Chairman of the Department, and I asked him:

"Excuse me, Sir! I am Peter Yellinek. I work for Dr. Dickerman, and I have been coming to the lectures and conferences for well over a year, but I still haven't received my appointment…"

The Chairman interrupted me with a quizzical look:

"Well, I noticed you here for a long time, but I don't remember receiving an application for your appointment. You should ask Dr. Dickerman to file it!"

In disbelief, I stood there with my mouth gaping, not knowing what to say. Finally, I mumbled:

"Thank you, Sir! I will ask Dr. Dickerman." That evening, I drove home feeling like a fool.

The next morning, I walked into Dr. Dickerman's office, greeted him, and immediately told him what had transpired the night before. For a long moment, he kept his gaze directed upward towards the ceiling, as if there was an answer to be found up there. Then he looked directly at me and firmly said:

"I know I spoke to the Chairman and filed an application for your appointment! He must have forgotten about it, or, I don't know, his secretary may have misplaced the application. But look! I definitely want you to get this appointment! I'll fill out a new application form and send it off right this morning! We'll get it in motion right away!"

I thanked him and went into my office. His words: "…right this morning," were still ringing in my ears, and instead of starting to work, I began calling all my friends from pathology residency training, those who were still working in and around NYC. I inquired if they knew of any suitable job openings in the City or suburbs. And Bingo! One of my friends from Columbia University told me of a vacancy that had just come up in a hospital affiliated with a medical school where he was currently doing research and teaching.

I called up, was asked to send in my resume, and within several days I was given an interview. It went very well. One week later, I received a contract for a position of Assistant Pathologist in diagnostic surgical pathology, with additional duties of leading the pathology residency training program and taking care of the histology laboratory. The position also carried the title of Assistant Professor of Pathology at the medical school, with opportunities to do research and give lectures to students. It sounded like an ideal position, exactly what I wanted. The pay was adequate, though it was a typical, low academic salary.

Overjoyed, I immediately signed the contract and mailed it back. The school had a large group of pathologists and doctoral scientists (PhDs) doing research. The Chairman of the Department and several senior members held large research grants, and the research suite of labs was equipped with three of the most modern electron microscopes.

The next day, as soon as I came to work, I handed Dr. Dickerman a nicely typed and signed letter of resignation. He acted with surprise, but immediately started imploring me to change my mind and stay on. He tried to persuade me with all kinds of arguments, but I just kept quiet. Then suddenly, he offered me an immediate raise in salary of 25 percent! I was taken aback by such an offer, but just kept looking at him without saying a word. Then he said:

"Please, think it over! Go home and sleep on it for a night or two. And think seriously about it!" and he handed back to me my letter of resignation. I said politely that I would think about it, but I knew right then that I would not accept his offer, even though the salary in my new academic position was going to be much lower than his proposal.

In fact, the sudden offer of a 25 percent raise in salary made me angry. I realized that not only did Dr. Dickerman neglect his promise of a medical school appointment, but for nearly two years, he kept me vastly underpaid. As he suggested, I did sleep one night on his generous offer. I slept well and satisfied, knowing that the next morning, I would make it clear in the nicest way that no amount of money could motivate me to remain in the current position.

The next day, as soon as I arrived at work, I entered Dr. Dickerman's office and handed him all anew my original letter of resignation. My explanation was short and to the point:

"I hope that you will understand, my principal interest is to work towards an academic career! I have just received an appointment at a medical school!"

"Well, my offer still stands!" he replied.

"Thank you, but I cannot accept it!" and I went into my office to begin with the daily work, happy and excited that in about one month, I would be starting to work in an academic position.

In assessing my situation, I had reason to be satisfied. My first job as an attending pathologist lasted barely two years, and during that time, I passed the specialty board exam, gained more experience in diagnostic pathology, and had good luck with my research on amyloid, the project I started while still in residency training. Working numerous evenings in the electron microscopy suite, I was constantly changing the method of tissue preparation until finally, one evening, the electron images on my fluorescent screen showed exactly what I had been searching for. I succeeded in obtaining, in the same field of view, amyloid particles in two different shapes, the filaments and the rings, and they were randomly mixed with one another. So, it appeared that amyloid had at least two different morphologic forms! I obtained pictures of good quality for publication. The riddle of amyloid ultra-structure was at least partly solved: if both forms represented amyloid, the conclusion was that it was a heterogeneous substance structured in more than one physical form. The high magnification achieved by electron microscopy was of no help in identifying the chemical composition or the origin of amyloid. The precise definition of amyloid would have to be done by other means.

I had written a paper describing my findings and had no trouble having it accepted in a reputable "reviewed journal". It was published in 1969. That small personal success took over five years of intermittent work, done mostly after regular work hours. I had to ask myself, what was the real value of this tiny contribution to science? It was minimal! It also showed that studying amyloid by electron microscopy was the wrong approach. The real nature of amyloid was still not known. A few years later, other researchers took a different approach and discovered by immunologic methods that amyloid represented a variety of small defective protein moieties appearing in different physical forms. Each form, depending on the organ of its origin, could be defined immunologically, and in some cases, the tiny amyloid moieties would be found circulating in the patient's blood and could be demonstrated by immunoelectrophoresis.

The greatest value I gained from engaging in research was that I learned the principles and the technique of electron microscopy. Along with that, I enjoyed the time spent in excitement and hopeful anticipation of a possible discovery. I also believed that publishing the paper about amyloid had a practical value; it helped me to receive the appointment of Assistant Professor, along with a new job at the medical school.

Chapter 4

The Draft Board

This story began one evening in the summer of 1968 when I came home from work, and Miriam handed me a letter from the draft board, an institution from which I have not heard in over five years. The fine people at the draft board sent me an unwelcome surprise. They advised me that I was "reclassified" from 5A to 1A, and therefore, that at 8 am, on such and such date, I must appear for an examination at the army recruiting station at 39 Whitehall Street, New York, NY.

I first heard of the existence of a "draft board" in 1962, a few months after Miriam and I disembarked at a midtown pier in NYC. One of my colleagues at the hospital where I worked as an intern, told me that, even though I was only an immigrant, I should get registered for the draft, which was compulsory for all healthy young men. Since no one told me about it at the point of immigration, I went to verify it with the hospital administration, and there I received the address and phone number of the local draft board. I was told that physicians were eligible for the draft till the age of 35, and I made an appointment for a visit to the local draft board. Within a few days, in December of 1962, I was registered and given a classification of 5A, which meant that I was past the draft age of 26. My physician status was not recognized, since I did not yet obtain a state license to practice medicine. In 1964, as soon as I passed the required examination and received a license to practice medicine in New York State, I immediately wrote to the draft board about my change of status.

The current notice from the draft board came at an inconvenient time. We had started a family; we had a one-year-old baby, and we were expecting our second child in the fall of 1968. Just then, the prospect of being drafted was not very convenient. The US was at the height of the Vietnam War, a war to which I never paid much attention, and the purpose of which I did not know. Why did the draft board not reclassify me to 1A and call me up in 1964, when I received the MD license and became eligible? A good friend gave me the simple answer to that question: because the Vietnam War started only in 1965.

On the day of my draft appointment, I left home very early in the morning and, instead of going to work, I drove into lower Manhattan to find a good parking space. In those days, one could still easily drive into Manhattan and find free parking on the street. While driving from our apartment in Scarsdale into NYC, I remembered that somewhere I'd already heard the name "Whitehall Street" but could not attach that memory to any specific item. I learned from the map that the location was far downtown, in the Wall Street area of Manhattan.

So, I arrived at 39 Whitehall Street Army Station just in time, a few minutes before 8 am. There was already a large group of young people slowly filing through the entrance door of an old building that had at least three or four floors. Inside were many spacious rooms with high ceilings, and in some of the rooms, there were large tables with chairs and many pens at the disposal of the visitors. In the reception area, I was registered, fingerprinted, photographed and given a bunch of sequentially numbered forms to fill out and hand in at correspondingly numbered windows. Filling out those forms took over an hour, and when I was done, I went to the nearest window that was free, window number four, and handed the clerk the form number four. The clerk took his time looking at some papers, then finally lifted his head, looked at me, and pushed my paper back toward me, yelling:

"Can't you read? Go first to window number one, there!" and he pointed with his finger and said:

"You have to hand in the forms exactly in order of numbers!" I just shrugged and said:

"OK, sorry!" The clerk gave me a dirty look and remarked:

"It looks like you will be the last one to finish here today!"

I looked around and saw that windows numbered 1 and 2 had long lines of men waiting. I found that an efficient way of submitting the forms, that is, by beginning at windows that were free did not work. The army procedure obviously did not allow acceptance of forms in any order other than the sequence of counting learned in grade school: 1, 2, 3, 4, so that form number 4 could in no way be submitted before form number 3. The army had an order established and designed to fit a perfect bureaucracy, and it was not meant to be subject to any change, neither for reason of efficiency, nor out of common sense.

An hour later, after having handed in the last of the forms, I was told to go to the second floor and report in the physical examination room. Having found the proper door, I entered a vast hall where about fifty young people stood, neatly lined up in three rows. All of them were standing up, with their pants dropped down on the floor. The sight appeared surreal! I was a little late and, apparently, the last one to join this group. I went to the back, to the end of the third row, quickly loosened my belt and let my pants drop to the floor. I did not want to be any different from the others. At one end of the hall, I saw a few men wearing white lab coats, probably doctors, nurses, or medical technologists. After a few minutes, a sharp voice announced:

"Now, y'all, lower your underpants and bend over!" and then, louder: "BEND OVER! ALL THE WAY!"

A doctor started walking behind the first row of naked, bent-over men, looking sharply into each backside and yelling loudly, in a crescendo manner:

"Cough! COUGH!" and then, "Harder! HARDER!"

Occasionally, a man would be asked for his name, which would be written down by the clerk following the doctor. *Aha*, I thought, *this one has hemorrhoids; he might be exempted.*

Standing at the very end of the third row of men, I had a perfect view of the entire hall. The scene before me was amusing: three rows of half-naked, mooning men! And in that very moment, it dawned on me where I first heard the name "Whitehall Street"; it was in a delightfully funny song, and right then, the sweet melody of it also popped into my head. It was an unforgettable tune, and its rhyming lyrics also began to resonate in my mind: "…inspected, detected, injected, infected, selected, neglected…" It was all about the very same army recruiting station where I was now being inspected! The song was called "Alice's Restaurant". As all this surged into my head, I got a terrible impulse to laugh. Whenever I observed something funny, a joyous laughter was an impulse that I found very hard to resist. I tried with all my power to suppress it, but just couldn't hold it back and burst out laughing. The sergeant at the end of the hall snapped in a sharp, menacing tone:

"QUIET! QUIIIEET! WHOO is that?"

I stopped instantly but with an extraordinary effort because I heard a few stifled guffaws around me. I was guilty and was caught, and I got a good yelling from the sergeant. My name was recorded, and it was not on account of any hemorrhoids. Together with my pants down and my bare ass I apologized, trying to sound as sincere as possible. It must have been to no avail because, even as I managed to stop laughing, I knew that my face was still red and contorted from the effort, and I wasn't able to straighten it fully. I just wore a guilty, crooked grin. *Now,* I thought, *I have been recorded in their "bad book", and there is a prospect of someday being sent to the farthest outpost in Vietnam, somewhere a thousand miles out from Saigon...* The doctor continued his ritual, examining the other draftees, and after he finished with all the backsides, there came a sharp order:

"Now y'all, stand up straight!"

The doctor started all anew, checking the men in the first row. This time, he walked in front of them and inspected their groins. He kept repeating: "Cough, COUGH!" all the while poking with his gloved fingers into the inguinal areas. Again, some names had to be recorded, and I knew those were the lucky owners of a hernia.

Next, we were ordered to pull up our pants and take off our shirts and undershirts. Then followed the inspection of various cavities and organs in our heads, and we were poked around our necks and armpits. Short squeals were heard; evidently, some men were ticklish. Again, more names were recorded, probably for swollen glands. Finally came the loud command:

"Now, get dressed!"

Then we had to go to another room to have our blood drawn. We also had to give some urine. Soon after that, an official came and loudly announced:

"Lunch time!" Then he started giving instructions: "Now, y'all go to mess-hall! Go out the building, turn right, and right again, 'round the corner and step down into the basement! Here are the tickets for the mess-hall!" and he pointed to a box on the table and added: "Be back at thirteen hours!"

Each of us picked up a meal ticket from the box and walked down towards the exit of the building. Somewhere along that morning, hearing how all others were responding, I learned to say loud and clear, "Yes, Sir!" instead of a resigned "OK".

I followed the trail of men walking out onto the street, turning around the corner, and then down the stairs into a basement. The mess hall was a large space with four rows of very long tables, and benches along each side. On one side of the hall was a line of men standing along a self-service food counter, and I joined them. The lunch was decent: two choices of entrees, a soup, a salad, and even a dessert with a choice of coffee or tea. I was not in the mood to eat, upset with the day's proceedings, and even more so by the thought that I might be called up for service. *What for? To serve in Vietnam?* With those thoughts, I ate some of the food, got up, took my tray, and went towards a broad kitchen window where the food trays were to be returned. Next to that window was a large metal barrel with a big sign above it: **"DIRTY DISHES"** and a black arrow pointing down to the barrel. I emptied my tray and put it on the kitchen window.

Suddenly, there appeared a man from behind the window and started roaring like a wounded beast. I could not understand a word of what he was saying, and I turned around to look behind me. *What is he screaming about?* Behind me, some of the men at the tables started getting up, and they were all looking at me. Then I understood one single word coming from the roaring man: "silver", and I got it! Among the dirty dishes, there was a single piece made of metal, the knife! All the rest, the forks, spoons, cups and plates, were made of disposable plastic. I had to find and fish out from the refuse the piece of "silver".

"Sorry", I said, putting the precious knife on the kitchen window. The shouting ended with a deep growl.

I walked lazily out onto the street and around the corner, back into the building to attend the afternoon session. I was depressed and miserable. The afternoon dragged on: there were more forms to be filled out. Some questions were about my past memberships in whatever clubs or political organizations and other activities, going back to the time of my adolescence! I was never a member of any political organization. I joined only sports clubs. Annoyed and bitter about all those questions, I wrote, "Do not remember". Anyway, those were the same questions I had to answer a year earlier on my application for citizenship, as if anyone was going to bother or be able to check the veracity of the answers!

Then I was sent to have chest X-rays, and that took quite a while. The technologist explained that instead of taking a few plate film images, they were using a movie camera. Film spools were smaller and easier to store. At least, there was some efficiency and common sense. Then came some more clerical procedures. By the time it was all finished, I felt exhausted. And, just as I was warned that morning, I was among the last people getting out of the building.

As for the result of the draft examination, I passed it and was confirmed as 1A, ready for service. Of course, the ready condition would exist till my 35th birthday, and that meant only a little over two years... Meanwhile, I found that most of my American-born colleagues had used certain known paths to avoid military service. Some of them joined the Berry Plan, by which they would be deferred until they finished their specialty training (residency), and only then could they be either drafted by a lottery system or would become free from the draft. Some joined the ROTC, which required that they attend regular short training sessions and meetings until the age of 35, instead of being called up for active duty. Some joined the Public Health services...

At that time, one of my friends, Subash R., also a pathologist, had recently accepted a job in Kingston, Ontario. Exhausted from the Whitehall Street experience, I took several days of vacation and drove up to visit Subash. From there, I proceeded to the beautiful city of

Toronto and stayed with yet another colleague. He introduced me to a group of his friends, and one of them invited me to join him and work at his hospital. That was nice, and I thanked him, but I would have to think about it… I returned home rested and relaxed.

Those two years, until my 35th birthday, I was living in the state of "ready for draft". It was a time occasionally marred by thoughts of uncertainty about the future… Days and months passed slowly, and Miriam and I enjoyed our two toddlers at home. Then came my 35th birthday, and we celebrated with old friends, having dinner at "La Crémaillère", an old French restaurant in Bedford, NY.

Later, when I described my Whitehall Street experience to some friends, the story was met with hearty laughter. One of them speculated that my laughing at the mooning men might have earned me a suspicion of being gay, and that might have been the reason why I was never called up. Another one said that there was a law that sole male survivors in a family had to be posted stateside, and the real need for physicians was overseas, in Vietnam. Several years later, I met a colleague who enjoyed the full benefit of that law. He was called up in 1968, during the height of the Vietnam War, but being the sole male survivor in his family, he spent his entire service time in the US.

Over following years, I remained in touch with my friends in Canada, and twelve years later, I again visited my friend Subash, who by then had moved with his wife and three sons back to the US and lived in Niagara Falls. One evening, at his house, we reminisced about the time when we were young enough to go to war…

Chapter 5

Harry

In the middle of 1969, I started working as an assistant pathologist in a hospital affiliated with a medical school in NYC. I first presented myself in the office of my immediate boss, the Chief of Surgical Pathology, Dr. Morton Braun. He welcomed me, and right away took me to Dr. Harry Knob, the other Assistant Pathologist, who would clue me in on all I needed to know about the operation of the department.

Harry was a friendly, middle-aged pathologist with whom I was to share all the diagnostic work in the department. Our offices were on the eighth floor of an old building and occupied a single, very large room with a twelve-foot ceiling and a seven-foot partition separating our two individual workspaces. Over that partition, we could hold a conversation, or one could hear if the other one was engaged on the phone. Harry was already ensconced in the slightly larger half of the room, with a desk, chair and a small sofa seat, and I got the space of my predecessor, the smaller half of the room, with a desk and chair facing a large window, through which I could see adjacent parts of our building and a piece the sky above. The office also had a large anteroom, furnished with a sofa and a small table for visitors, and a sink with a long counter space that held the equipment for frozen sections of tissues submitted for rapid diagnosis. Two chairs and a table with a large double-headed microscope for diagnostic sign-out conferences and consultations were situated by the front edge of our office partition.

Harry had been working in that office for several years, and on that first day, he explained to me the entire flow of work in the department and then introduced me to the clerical staff in the office, the technicians in the histology lab, and the residents in training. A tall, robust fellow with thinning reddish hair, he was lively and pleasant, moving his whole body and gesticulating while talking. He reminded me of a bouncing teddy bear. Usually smiling, he spoke with a Chicago accent and a slight lisp. Right on, Harry let me know that he loved to do the diagnostic work but had little interest in teaching and no interest in research. Within the next few days, Harry also provided me with all essential information about the clinicians on the medical staff, particularly the surgeons, gynecologists, oncologists, and dermatologists, all of those who provided most of the material for our diagnostic work.

When I asked why the pathologist, who previously held my position, left, Harry only said that it was a young lady who resigned rather suddenly and took a job as director of pathology in a small hospital across town.

About six months later, as Harry got to know me a little better, one day at lunch, he quietly proceeded to tell me in great confidence, why that lady pathologist resigned. It turned out that our immediate boss, Dr. Braun, had been passionately enamored with her for several years. He kept carrying on, pursuing her, trying to court her and caress her. Dr. Braun even wrote love poems dedicated to the young lady. Whenever he found her in a room alone, he would grope her and try to kiss her. It had apparently become an open secret within the confines of the department. Harry concluded the story by saying:

"She couldn't take it anymore and found another job!"

Harry was still in touch with that pathologist, and he eventually introduced me to her. At that the time, she needed part-time help in the clinical laboratory, and she offered me a part-time position as Director of Clinical Laboratory, with the duty of checking the lab 3 to 4 times a week. I was glad to accept that position and do a little moonlighting to bolster my academic salary. That job gave me a chance to get acquainted with the meaning of "turf" in the field of medicine. That turf had to do with the politics regarding blood bank services in NYC. I discovered that my New York State Certificate of Director of Laboratory was perfectly valid in NYC, except when it came to directing a blood bank. The NYC Department of Health required that a State certified pathologist take a separate City directed examination, to be approved as a "Director of Blood Bank".

I obtained the required application forms from the City office, paid the fees, and after a few weeks, received an invitation to take the test for the Blood Bank Director's certification. First, there was a written test given at an office of the NYC Department of Health, and I passed it with a high score. Then, there was a second part of the exam, an oral test, again to be taken by appointment at the same office. At the oral test, I was introduced to four examiners, all of them specialists in internal medicine with a subspecialty in hematology. Each examiner posed a hypothetical question by describing a made-up patient problem convoluted by several complicating factors, all of them leading to more than one solution… There was no chance that anyone could fathom what was aimed at, other than to create confusion. One of the questions was so long and involved that the examiner took over two minutes to fully describe all the tangential complications. When he ended, I politely asked if he would not mind repeating the question because, I said, "I did not hear well all the details". Of course, the examiner could not repeat his longwinded convolutions, but proceeded to give a different version… Well, I tried to answer each examiner's question as best I could.

About a week later, I received a letter from the NYC Department of Health informing me that I had failed the oral exam. Then I found that most hospital blood banks in NYC were run by hematologists, and only exceptionally few were directed by a pathologist. The City had a large group of hematologists who considered blood banks as their own 'turf'. They had enough political influence to insinuate themselves as examiners for the test, even though clinical pathologists had more training in blood compatibility testing than did the internists. I decided to prepare very thoroughly for a repeat oral test by reading about all the new developments in the blood bank area. I took the repeat oral test and again failed in the same manner as the first time.

I then wrote a sharp letter to the City commissioner responsible for licensing of blood banks, describing the oral test as a "kangaroo court" composed exclusively of internists/hematologists, who acted with the intent of keeping the pathologists out of the blood banks. The letter was never answered. Six weeks later, when I called the commissioner's office and insisted on speaking directly to her, I was told that the commissioner was in the process of reviewing my case and would "soon respond" to my inquiry.

About two months later, when my regular annual renewal of NYC lab director's certificate arrived in the mail, I had a very pleasant surprise. Along with chemistry, hematology, microbiology, and serology, the certificate included the blood bank! I framed and kept that certificate for many years, even after I stopped practicing in NYC.

I noticed that Harry spent a lot of his free time reading newspapers or being on the phone with his broker. It appeared that the stock market was one of his passions, and it seemed as if it were an addiction. He tried to introduce me to "the market", proposing one or another "excellent opportunity" for investment. He came to me one day, all excited, and said: "Look, here is a start-up company called Ecology.

It's here in Brooklyn, and it has a great future! It will collect garbage from all over the City and convert it into fuel! My broker recommends it highly, and I already bought into it."

I made it clear to Harry that I was not at all in a position to make investments. I had to save every penny for a downpayment on a house. Anyway, I did not know anything about the stock market. I grew up and got an education amidst a crumbling communist economy, far from any stock market or exposure to financial entrepreneurship. The stock market was to me like a forest full of ghosts to a four-year-old child. I told Harry that I trusted the stock market as much as I believed in Alchemy, the medieval pseudoscience that claimed it was possible to transform ordinary metals into gold… It took a long time before I learned that, at least for some people and under certain circumstances, the stock market could have a positive effect.

Harry was a patient and persistent man, and he kept trying to educate me on financial matters. Every now and then, he would inform me about some "great new deal coming up" and how the market was "bullish". He explained what exactly the "bull market" meant, and at that, he also introduced me to the meaning of the "bear market". This prompted me one day to ask:

"And how did these animals get into the stock market?"

"It all began many years ago, during the gold rush. There was, at the time, a stock market in San Francisco, and people in that area, out West, used to entertain themselves by watching a contest, a fight between a bull and a bear. They would dig a deep, square pit in the ground and lower into it a bull and then the bear, and they would watch them fight to death."

"This is gory. I wouldn't want to see it."

"Nor would I, but never mind! The point is, when the bull fights, he crouches down and hits with his head moving up, trying to gore the bear with his horns, and that's why "bullish" means the market is moving up!"

"And, what about the 'bear market'?"

"Well, the bear fights standing tall, and he tries to claw the bull with his paws, hitting down."

"So, 'bearish' means that the market is going down. I guess, you believe that in those fights, the bull usually won?"

"I don't know, but it could be."

"Well, right now, I really don't care to get involved in the market nor with any of these beasts."

"But, I think, someday you will!"

Harry was a true believer in "the market", and he never ceased to talk about it.

At one point, Harry happily informed me that his stock portfolio had grown to well over one million dollars. It was in the seventies a nice bundle for a person in his early forties. I congratulated him, but still would not be persuaded to invest in any stock. Unfortunately, soon thereafter, the market suffered a significant "correction". To make a greater gain while the market was still rising, Harry bought many shares "on margin", borrowing 90 percent of the purchase price from his broker, and put up as collateral his entire portfolio. As the price of those shares suddenly dropped below the purchase price, the broker asked for margin purchases to be fully paid, and the required funds were obtained by selling the largest part of Harry's portfolio unfortunately, at a loss. About three-quarters of Harry's first million were wiped out.

Then Harry admitted that buying shares on margin was a mistake, and he said he would never do it again. He also explained that the market may sometimes act in an unpredictable manner. A war or any other economic calamity could throw it off its bullish course. However, he was confident that the market would recover and again begin to rise. To prove it, he showed me a chart of the market's past performance. That chart looked like a seesaw, with lots of fluctuation, although it did show an upward trend until the current drop. The worst calamity was that after losing most of his money, Harry became noticeably depressed. Not long after that, he suffered a small heart attack. He spent one week in the hospital, and after recovering for another week at home, he came back to work.

Within a month, he was fully recovered, apparently cheerful and again bouncing around like a teddy bear. And soon I could hear him behind our partition, again with great élan, murmuring to his broker on the phone… About a year later, Harry let me know that the very promising start-up company, "Ecology", had become a "penny stock" after a brief rise in value. I learned another market term which described a supposedly "good idea" that, unfortunately, "went south". While working alongside Harry, aside from expanding my experience in the practice of pathology, I also received some education in the stock market and its vocabulary.

With Harry's frequent talk about the "market", I wanted to get informed from some other sources and began to read about it on my own. The stock market presented a morass of numbers, laws, opportunities and traps, like a game, where the rules were fuzzy and the outcomes dubious. With its up and down movements, it appeared like an alluring but inscrutable competition. In reality, it was not very different from gambling. Looking closer, one could see that big gains were made either by people who had the "inside knowledge" or tips, or on very rare occasions plain luck. Then there were also professional traders who gambled with other people's money and got rich on trade commissions. The few people who had a profound understanding of a specific sector of the economy were able to make a profit consistently. It is possible that anyone might get a good insight into the stock market by careful observation of the movement of a particular stock (or a group of stocks in an industry, e.g. pharmaceutical) and then make money 'buying low' and 'selling high'. However, that approach required lots of time and patience, reading political and economic news and keenly watching the dumb, boring price movements without an end. Who would want to spend his life that way? Perhaps a person whose main passion is driven by nothing but a strong desire for money, wanting more and ever more of it. The broad masses of people use the stock market by haphazardly following one or another advice, and their chances of making a profit are as likely as winning a lottery. For most people, the stock market is nothing but a game of gambling. Besides that, I remembered that while visiting Europe in 1966, one US dollar was worth four German marks, but then, in 1975, it was worth only 2.4 marks. There was the inflation, and the whole world was subject to it, although to a variable degree.* The rise in the

---

* Having observed the inflation over many years, I noticed that there was a substantial difference between the officially published inflation figure and the actual rise of retail prices. It seems that the official inflation is calculated by averaging the prices of raw, unfinished products: oil, copper, steel, cotton, corn, soybeans, etc. When people go to buy the finished products, which are sold in retail (gasoline, groceries, clothing, or pay for school tuition and other services), all these items show an annual price increase that is about double the official inflation rate. College tuitions have, over the years, seen annual inflation of more than 8-10 percent. Inflation is also a reason why today workers' wages have a lower purchasing power than fifty years ago. On the other hand, aiming to keep up with inflation, the annual incomes of corporate CEOs, CFOs and other executives have grown to be many times higher than wages of workers. The purchasing power of CEO's income is now higher than it was fifty years ago.

"market" is expressed by ever-higher dollar numbers, which give an illusion of great gain. However, due to inflation, the real value of the stocks has increased relatively little as the dollar's purchasing power has become lower. Thus, inflation reduces the actual value of gains on the stock market, and in addition, capital gains are subject to taxation.

After having observed the odd realm of the "market", I decided to invest my savings conservatively, only in relatively safe treasury bonds, and I would stay away from gambling with the stocks. Despite the difference in our interests outside the office, Harry and I got along very well. We helped each other in our work, and we became good friends, enjoying each other's company. Harry was a pleasant and warm person, and in professional work, he was a wise and level-headed companion. When we had a difficult case with a doubtful diagnosis, we would first consult with one another and then submit it to our immediate boss, Dr. Braun, for a final decision. There were only very few, rare cases in our practice where all three of us could not come up with a definitive diagnosis. Then we would send the microscopic slides to a renowned expert in the specific subject, and that way, we would usually get a conclusive diagnosis. At that time, expert opinions and consultations were given gratis, as a matter of courtesy, and no pathologist would ever send a bill for such services. A 'difficult case' presented a challenge that we gladly accepted, because it took us away from the relatively monotonous routine. On those rare occasions, we always went to see the patient in person to get a complete medical history directly from the source. And in some cases, just a more thorough history of illness would direct us to the right diagnosis.

Here is an example gleaned from those interesting, rare cases where we had to seek help from expert consultants. One day at the sign-out conference, a senior resident presented a tumor of the ovary that looked different from anything I had ever seen before. When neither one of us within our department could come up with a plausible diagnosis, it was decided to mail out copies of microscopic slides to two expert consultants, one at Cancer Memorial Hospital in NYC and the other at MD Anderson Hospital in Texas. A request for a pathologic consultation must always include a full, thorough history of the patient, and so I went to investigate. The patient was a 14-year-old girl who was admitted to the emergency room following a sudden onset of abdominal pain and vaginal bleeding. To the great surprise of the girl's mother, the emergency room physician diagnosed pregnancy at term. The girl was about to deliver a baby. The patient was extremely obese, and her mother never suspected that she was pregnant. The baby was delivered stillborn, and after delivery, the obstetrician found that there was still a very large mass in the abdomen, and it was not a twin baby. With consent from the mother, the girl was operated on, and a very large tumor of the left ovary was taken out. More than two weeks later, the consultant from MD Anderson Hospital informed us that the girl had one of those extremely rare malignant tumors that have been described only six or seven times in the whole medical literature. The other consultant made the diagnosis of a "malignant tumor of unknown type". During my remaining years at the hospital, that patient was not seen again, and we never got a follow-up.

Nearly every month at work, there was some event that interrupted our routine. One morning, Harry came in all disheveled, staggering into the office with a torn jacket and broken glasses. He sat on his sofa and let out a sigh.

"Harry, what happened to you?" I asked.

"I was mugged! Just a few minutes ago, I was coming out of the subway, and two guys pushed me against the wall! They took my watch and wallet and ran away. I had only about ten dollars of cash. That's all they got…"

"Well, it's good, they did not hurt you! Go now, wash your face, and you'll be fine!"

The next day, when Harry came in, he showed me a new little gadget. He bought a spray gun with mace and said he would keep it in his pocket, to always be ready.

That little gadget created an interesting phenomenon a few months later during an inspection of our department by the NYC Department of Health. There were two inspectors, and as we followed them from room to room, each room seemed to have a strange, unpleasant odor that we could not explain. The inspectors were puzzled, and we assured them that we never encountered that odor before and had no idea where it came from. When my eyes began smarting, I realized that Harry, being tense about the inspection, unconsciously kept squeezing on the mace in his pants pocket.

Before we moved to the next room, I told him quietly, to take his hand out of the pocket. As we moved on, the odor was no longer with us, and the inspectors never found the source of it. When the inspection was over, Harry and I had a good laugh over the leaking mace. During the six years that we worked together, Harry was mugged one more time, and again, he only lost his wallet with a few dollars in it, and a cheap Timex watch. He was not hurt because, fortunately, it happened so fast that he never had a chance to use the spray.

Harry had a steady girlfriend who would occasionally come to visit in the late afternoon, sit on the sofa in our anteroom, and wait for him to finish work. Her name was Kristin, and she was a young, tall, well-built woman who was very pleasant and always wore a smile. Our office secretaries nicknamed her "The Go-Go-Girl". Harry had been going out with Kristin for several years, and they were talking about marriage, but there was a problem. Harry lived in a suburban apartment together with his widowed father, who was very religious and was adamantly opposed to this marriage on account of Kristin's religion. Harry was Jewish, and he came from a very orthodox family, while Kristin was a Lutheran. She was willing to convert, but for Harry's father, that would not be good enough. Harry was in all his tastes entirely secular, but he loved and respected his father very much, and so, the marriage was put in abeyance. Kristin had a little apartment in NYC, and their life together was quite comfortable.

Harry had a curious habit: once a week, after finishing work, he would go to the animal department in the research building and take a little mouse to bring it home. When I asked him what the mouse was for, he explained that his father was allergic to animal fur, and he kept at home a pet reptile, a small python, only three feet long. He praised the python as being very clean and undemanding. Speaking of it, he said:

"…eats only one live mouse per week and makes only one dry pellet. You can watch him chase the mouse and swallow him in one gulp, and then you see a bulge, slowly moving through his body…"

One day, Harry told me that the python had caused a little shock to a friend of his. The python had a habit of disappearing somewhere in the apartment for a day or two, usually hiding in a closet. As a visiting friend was leaving the apartment and putting on his overcoat, he had a hard time putting his arm through the sleeve. Suddenly, out of the sleeve slithered the python, and his friend had quite a fright. Of course, it all ended well. The python acted more scared than the owner of the coat.

When Harry's father passed away, he and Kristin decided to move to California to be near his younger brother who had a house in L.A. Harry resigned, and after he left, I missed him very much. The young assistant pathologist hired into Harry's position was very diligent, correct and respectful, but he lacked the spirit, the wit and the humor that I enjoyed with Harry. I missed a certain deeper understanding, maybe a generational connection. Besides, Harry was not only a colleague and partner with whom I shared the daily work, but he had become a real friend. Separated by great distance, we both were busy in our own worlds, and slowly, we began to lose touch.

The first time Harry called me from L.A., he gave me the good news: he passed the California state medical exam and found a good job. Kristin and he were married, and they lived in a nice apartment, occasionally visited with Harry's brother's family, and were hoping to start a family of their own. We called each other every few months and stayed abreast with our little news. About two years after he left, Harry called me early one evening, and his voice was hardly audible. Clearly, something was wrong. He told me he was in a hospital, recovering from a heart attack. I tried to encourage him, but he complained that he was convalescing very slowly and was desperately depressed. So, I said:

"Oh, come on, Harry, you are still young! Just take it easy, and you'll get well! You'll be fine! Tell me: how is Kristin?"

"Peter! Something terrible has happened!" Harry paused and then continued: "A week ago, I came home from work and found Kristin dead! She committed suicide! I found her lying on the floor of our bedroom with her head shattered... I kept in our apartment a gun, and Kristin took it and fired it into her mouth! And she left no note... Then, soon, I felt the heart attack, and the pain was so sharp that I could barely call my brother... I don't know why she did it! Why? Why? I don't know, and I will never know it... We were so happy..."

"Oh, Harry! I am so sorry, so sorry! These things have no answer!"

"In a few days… they will be discharging me from the hospital. I hate the thought of going home… I don't know what I am going to do…"

"Harry, go to your brother and stay awhile with his family, try to spend some time with them! Get to know your two nephews! I know it's difficult, but you are not a quitter! You'll get through…" and we spoke for another few minutes. In the end, he promised to spend some time at his brother's house.

The next time I spoke to Harry was about two weeks later. He was staying at his brother's house, was again working, and was ready to go back to his apartment and have it put in order. I was glad that he appeared out of his depression and was even thinking of taking a little vacation.

About two months later, one evening, there was a phone call, and I heard a man with a deep raspy voice:

"Hello! I am Dave Knob, Harry's brother. Harry often talked about you. Last week he suffered another heart attack, and all along, it looked like he was going to pull through. Only yesterday, he said he was going to call you… but during last night… he passed away. He was only 51…"

"I am so sorry! He was such a dear man and my good friend. I will never forget our years of friendship! I am so sorry!"

"Thank you!"

"Goodbye…" I hung up, feeling a ball in my throat, and there was nothing more I would be able to say. He probably felt the same. Every now and then, the fond memory of Harry pops into my head, and I remember with pleasure how the two of us worked side-by-side, how we talked, sometimes over the partition, and how we enjoyed our warm and understanding friendship and humor.

Chapter 6

The Union

A part of my duty at the medical school hospital involved supervision of the histology laboratory that prepared all our microscopic slides. That lab had a staff of six technologists: five women, including the lead technologist, and one man, all scheduled to work from 6:30 am to 2:30 pm. That lab was the place where I first became aware of a hospital union. It came out one day when the lead technologist, a lady in her fifties, came to my office with a complaint. She claimed that the man on her team did not do any work! She said that, day after day, the man would show up in the morning, put on his lab coat, and declare that he had to go attend union meetings and some other union business. He would come back into the lab after lunch, about half an hour before the end of the workday, when most of the day's chores had been completed by the other five technologists. She said the man was a union official, a "shop steward". It was a title I was not at all familiar with, but it seemed as though a shop steward's only job was to attend union meetings.

Compelled to investigate it, I first visited the office of the Personnel Department (the term HR was invented later) to inform myself about the union and the work rules concerning union officials. There, I received a few sheets with written rules, procedures and instructions on what to do in case of infractions at work. Following instructions, I left a message in the histology lab for the technologist to come to my office as soon as he appears in the lab. Meeting him, I gave him a formal "verbal admonishment" about his duty to do a fair share of work in the lab, exactly as stated in the personnel protocol. He explained that as a "shop steward", he had the right to attend union meetings but promised to spend more time helping in the lab.

Thereafter, the lead technologist reported to me that the man had helped in the lab for about one hour a day, and he had been absent the rest of the time. I proceeded to follow the personnel procedure, and I served the shop steward with a second admonition, this time in writing, including a warning that if he were to receive a third admonition, he could be dismissed. After that, the man started to participate in lab work much more, reportedly about four hours per day. At that point, the leader of the histology team told me that she was afraid of the man, as he exhibited some threatening behavior, and she preferred not to make any further complaints. I was satisfied that the problem was resolved as well as it could be…

Several weeks after this little incident, I received a certified letter from the federal district court addressed to my work address. It was a notice of a lawsuit brought against me by the shop steward, who accused me of "discrimination based on color". Reading it, at first, I felt very upset and angry. My procedure regarding his work habits was executed exactly according to the rules received from the personnel office, and it was done for a valid reason. All I knew of him was that he was an immigrant from Haiti and a technologist who did not fulfill his work obligations. I also knew that he behaved with female co-workers in a verbally offensive and threatening manner, an additional problem that I did not choose to address. The skin color of this technologist was no darker than mine in summer when I was well-tanned. We both were equally brown. I had to calm down, and I folded the letter, put it in my bag, and went on with my work. I would read the letter again later in the evening, at home.

After carefully reading the court letter for a second time, I called a close friend and read it to him. He asked me a few questions about what exactly happened between the plaintiff and me. He said that, even though I was acting correctly, a lawsuit of this kind was a serious matter, and he advised me to immediately hire a good attorney, or I could give the letter to the hospital administration, and their attorney might take care of it. I called a couple more friends, and they gave me similar advice. Then I remembered that even though all my ancestors resided in Europe for nearly two thousand years, in the US, I was easily taken for a person of color. I became aware of it a few years earlier, after having received the US citizenship. It appears that in US, the European immigrants with darker skin complexion, usually those from the southern Mediterranean area, may be considered as 'brown' or 'colored'.

A few years earlier, when I visited the office of the Immigration Service to be examined for admission to US citizenship, I noticed that the examining officer had crossed out something and then put a new checkmark on my application. At the time, I did not know what he did, and I did not pay much attention to it. But three months later, when I received my citizenship certificate, I found that I was in a "mixed marriage"! Apparently, the immigration officer had crossed out the checkmark "fair" for my skin color and then put a checkmark elsewhere. The immigration examination was in August when I was deeply tanned. My skin was indeed quite brown, my hair was jet black and curly, and the officer, seeing me face to face, did his job, either according to instructions or just by his personal inclination. That happened at the end of 1967, when, after five long years of waiting, I was happy to finally obtain US citizenship. At that time, the assessment of my skin color meant only that my "interracial marriage" might not be legal in every state of US. Now, suddenly, my officially declared skin color became very convenient.

I went to the bank, pulled out of the safe my "naturalization certificate", looked at it, and decided that I did not need to ask for help from any lawyer. I wrote a letter back to the federal court, simply stating that the accusation against me was without foundation since I, myself, was a colored person, as stated in my citizenship certificate. Within a few weeks, I received a notice from the court indicating that the lawsuit against me was dismissed.

With all that, I became more cognizant that my skin was neither white nor "fair". My skin in winter could be best described as "olive" or "swarthy", and in summer, it becomes so well-tanned that my color is indistinguishable from that of an African American of mixed blood. I always believed that a person represents, whatever other people may see with their own eyes. Apparently, my personal appearance gives a perception of a "brown" person, especially to those who pay great attention to the color of skin. I am certainly not a "Caucasian". * My European origin is Mediterranean, and if one goes back by two millennia, my ancestors came from the southeast side of that sea, near

---

* The term "Caucasian", that common euphemism for people of "fair" or "white" complexion, always grated me the wrong way. Caucasus is a mountain on the border between Asia and Europe, and the so-called "Caucasian" people did not come from that mountain. Why is it that in the US, only people of color are called with an adjective, like: 'African Americans', or 'Latin Americans', or 'Japanese Americans' and 'Chinese Americans', etc.? Why do we not hear of 'European Americans'?? I have the impression that the term "Caucasian" was invented by people who believe that "white skin" is the most important characteristic of humans. Those are the same people who believe that "might is right", that muscle is more important than brain, and that they have a right to rule and take from "others" or destroy "them…" The term "Caucasian" evokes thoughts of the proponents of racism. Then one remembers that the US Immigration Act of 1924 put severe restrictions on immigration quotas of darker-skinned people from Southern and Eastern Europe. It is a sad fact that racism is deeply ingrained in human culture, and most of it starts with the upbringing of children… Once they grow up, the racists do not willingly respond to friendly treatment, and they often resist the law. The sad truth is, that racism is an affliction that may be found in all humans, no matter whether their skin is white, yellow, brown, black, red or green.

the border of Asia and Africa. Henceforth, on the census forms and other similar documents inquiring about my race, I always check the box for "Other", and in the open space for race, I write: "Human". To belong to the human race is, for me, good enough, although sometimes, it is hard to tell whether the humans are better than some species of rapacious beasts.

To go back to the unions: the only other experience I had with the hospital union was on occasions when our pathology offices needed some repair. The offices were in an old building, and the need for various repairs was frequent. Each time we called the engineering department to fix a problem, at least two men would come up to offer help. For example, when an electrical outlet was dead, invariably, two electricians would show up. One time, the outlet was in the very corner of my office, and no more than one person could come close to it. Of course, one of the two electricians changed the outlet with a new one, while the second man patiently stood by the entry door and waited for the job to be completed. Such scenes were repeated on numerous occasions.

Sometimes, while witnessing the repair work, I would engage the second electrician in a light, friendly conversation. I noticed that he had a familiar accent, and I found that he was an immigrant from Yugoslavia. I told him that I, too, was from the same country and even from the same province, Croatia. Afterwards, that man sometimes used to come up during his lunch break and knock on the door of my office. He craved to exchange a few words in his native tongue. He was lonely. He alone escaped from communist Yugoslavia at the age of 17, came to the US, and became a licensed electrician. His whole family remained in a small town in Dalmatia, and he was supporting them. His father was very ill; in fact, he was dying of liver cancer. The electrician told me that many people in his town and in the surrounding region had liver cancer and some other types of cancer or leukemia. He was from the town of Dugi Rat, and I was familiar with that town. It housed a large plastics factory built in Yugoslavia right after the Second World War, and it made PVC (polyvinyl chloride).

As a physician, I knew that vinyl chloride was a highly toxic, cancer-causing agent, and the communist government of Yugoslavia did not bother to install any protective devices for the workers, nor did it let them know that working in that factory was dangerous. It was the usual disregard for human life practiced by communist dictatorships and, in many instances, also by some "democracies". I told the electrician to warn his family not to ever work in that factory. When his father passed away, he came to see me and let me know that the rest of his family had moved out of that town because, for years, the air in the area was full of fumes from the factory, and one could easily recognize the acrid smell.

One day, the same electrician came to my office, visibly upset. He wanted to tell me something, but was hesitant, till I encouraged him by saying:

"Look, I can see that something is bothering you. You may tell me! I am a doctor and a friend; you don't have to be afraid."

"Well, yes, but you must not tell this to anyone. You know, there is a group of us, Croats, here in the City, and we all escaped from communism in Yugoslavia. We meet regularly in our little club to sing our homeland songs and to eat our kind of food and speak our language."

"That sounds nice!"

"Yes, but there was a problem! Mate, my best friend from Croatia said something… something about the Serbs, that some of them were good people, and that we should not hate all Serbs. In the evening, after we parted, out on the street, in the dark, Mate was caught by several of our Croat members and was beaten very, very badly and left lying on the sidewalk. He had many broken bones and is now still in the hospital. I heard from his wife, and I visited him. When he gets out, he says he will move to another state. He is scared to remain in this city…" and he fell silent.

"Well, you must be very careful what you say at your club; they know that you are a friend of Mate."

"Yes, and Mate's wife is Serbian!"

I only nodded, and we understood each other.

This sad little story shows that aside from racism, humans also suffer from deep ethnic hatred and intolerance. This occurred in the mid-seventies, a time when organized groups of Croat immigrants were committing such acts that the US government designated them as terrorists. There was an incident of hijacking of a commercial airplane over Chicago, with a demand to announce over public media Croat nationalist grievances against the Yugoslav government. Then there was an armed attack on the Yugoslav consulate in NYC and a massive bombing of La Guardia Airport, all events perpetrated by Croats who belonged to a nationalist group called Ustashe, formerly associated with Nazis. Those Croats carried their hatred and fights with Serbs all the way to the US, and the same status has not changed even today, fifty years later.

It was only after I got to know the pair of hospital electricians quite well, that one day I dared to ask them why the two of them always showed up for every small repair that could be done by one person.

"It's the rule! It's the union!" one of them answered dryly, and they made no further comment. Obviously, they did not want to talk about that subject. What this rule was achieving was left to my imagination.

I knew that electrical workers were well paid, and this union rule opened an opportunity for the creation of more jobs and the appearance that the union provided more work.

As for the unions in general, I found it disturbing to read frequent articles in the press describing the behavior of union "bosses", the teamster's affairs, the disappearance of their top leader, etc. - news of unsavory taste. With all that, my personal experience with unions, though limited, was unfortunately molded in a negative way. I felt that the unions had a positive role for workers in mining, trucking, large factories, and similar manufacturing or agricultural industries. A medical institution, a hospital, where sick people need help, compassion, and understanding, I felt, was not suited for the manner of action practiced by rule of members of a workers' union.

Chapter 7

Moonlighting

Already during the residency training, many of my colleagues used to have a second job, usually in the evenings or at night. They were "moonlighting". It was a source of additional income, especially for those who had a family with children. A few worked making house calls as general practitioners, others did autopsies in small hospitals or in nursing homes, and some worked as "house physicians", covering night shifts in private hospitals. At the time, in the sixties, doctor's visits were paid in cash, and making house calls was somewhat dangerous. While visiting a walk-up apartment, physicians were occasionally attacked and robbed.

As did most of my fellow residents, I, too, engaged in moonlighting. I preferred to do night shifts, serving as a house physician in a small private hospital. The latter job involved doing a history and physical examination on all newly admitted patients and, when needed, dispensing medications for sleep or pain. The job was easy: for the largest part of the night, one could rest in the on-call room without being disturbed. It was also well paid: if I worked four nights per month, the earnings equaled three months of the salary I received as a resident in pathology.

One of those nights, working as a house physician, I experienced an event that is hard to forget. I was awakened in the middle of the night by a call to come and see a patient in the emergency room. There, I saw a young woman who complained of severe bleeding, lasting for the last several hours. She gave a history of having had four days earlier a gynecologic curettage in the same hospital. I examined her and found considerable bleeding, and it was clear that to stop the bleeding, she would have to be admitted to the hospital and have another, more thorough curettage. The emergency room nurse informed me that every admission to the hospital had to be first cleared with the hospital owner, a gynecologist who lived in Westchester County, NY. As required, I picked up the phone and called the owner.

Hearing the story, he immediately remembered the patient by name and then told me very sharply:

"Do not admit her! Send her to another hospital! She still owes me money for previous visits, and she never paid for the curettage she had a few days ago."

"Dr. X, how can I send her away? She is bleeding, quite a significant amount…" He cut me off, screaming angrily:

"Now, listen! You just woke me up! And I just told you what to do!" and he hung up.

This physician and owner of a small hospital knew how to give orders! I was upset, but I still had to think and make a choice: what to do… I calmed down and gathered some more information. The patient lived very near the hospital and had simply walked to the emergency room. She had no means of transportation, and according to the nurse, at 3 am, it was not possible to obtain a taxi in that neighborhood. The nearest public City Hospital that would admit her was more than a mile away. Despite the owner's order, I felt it was mandatory to admit the patient into the hospital, keep her under observation till morning, and then do a procedure to stop the bleeding. I had the patient formally admitted, wrote up her chart, and went back to the on-call room. In the morning, I gave my night report to the day shift physician and left for my regular work as resident in pathology.

That same morning at work, the pathology office secretary called me to take a phone call from Dr. X., the owner of the private hospital. As soon as I picked up the phone and identified myself, he started yelling:

"You are fired! You will not get paid for last night! That will teach you to…" The rest I did not hear because I slowly lowered the receiver into the cradle of the phone. Jenny, the polite British office secretary looked at me with an expression of surprise. She noticed that I did not end the call in the proper way, with a greeting. I felt obliged to explain:

"Well… did you hear the screaming coming from the other end?" She nodded.

"Thanks for the call!"

Walking out of her office, I thought to myself, *to hell with that gynecologist! I can always find a job in another hospital, hopefully with a more ethical owner...*

Then there was another moonlighting opportunity, and yet another experience to remember. One evening, a few years later, during my first job as an attending pathologist, I received a call from Dr. Harvey, a senior pathologist from the medical school. He asked me if I would be interested in replacing him in a position at a large private nursing home in the Bronx. The home had a small clinical laboratory which needed a director, with weekly visits and on rare occasions, there was an autopsy. According to the contract at my principal job, I was allowed to do any private work outside of my regular hours, and I accepted Dr. Harvey's offer. He gave me more detailed information about the job and directed me to contact and meet with the administrator of the nursing home.

Very soon, I submitted my resume and was interviewed by the administrator and the Medical Board of the nursing home, and two weeks later, I received a letter from the Board President, informing me that I was accepted for the position of Director of Laboratory. The letter also instructed me to set up a meeting with the administrator to discuss my salary and to sign a contract. A day later, Dr. Harvey called me at work:

"Hello Peter! I just got in the mail a copy of your appointment. Congratulations! We should meet and talk about it as soon as you can!"

"Yes, Dr. Harvey, and I thank you very much!"

"You are welcome, Peter! There is still an issue that I would rather not discuss over the phone."

"I am sure no one is listening. Please, go ahead! You are on a direct line to my office."

"Well… you know… we have to discuss my compensation."

"Your compensation…" and it flashed through my mind that he wanted me to pay him for letting me take over his job. "…when you asked me if I was interested in the position, you did not say anything about the compensation! But please, tell me, what would you like?"

He started hemming and hoeing, and finally mumbled something about "the customary fee" that was due to him for the favor of letting me have the job. He explained that I would be enjoying the benefits of that salaried position for a long time. Finally, upon further prodding, he came out with the figure and asked for the equivalent of a year's salary and said we'd have to meet within the next few days so I could pay him in cash. Being completely inexperienced in such dealings, I was both baffled and repulsed by his demand. In an instant, I felt that the whole deal wasn't worth it, and I would not pay any "customary fee". I simply told him:

"No, Dr. Harvey! I am not used to paying such fees. Maybe someone else… I thank you for the offer." and I hung up, quite disappointed.

That conversation and that whole proposition left me with a bad taste, but I soon forgot about it. About three weeks later, I received a phone call from the administrator of the nursing home. He reminded me that we still had to meet to discuss my remuneration and sign the contract. Dr. Harvey, he said, was expected to leave town within the next two weeks… So, I understood that Dr. Harvey had just let it go, and I did get that part-time position.

The job turned out to be well compensated, and it was easy and undemanding. I kept it for the next nine years, until I moved out of the metropolitan area and gave the job to a pathologist who was an old friend. During those nine years, I also periodically held other moonlighting positions that lasted anywhere from several months to a year. Suffice it to say that without moonlighting jobs and with an academic salary, there would have been a much longer time before I could afford a house for our family.

Throughout the first ten years of my employment as an attending pathologist, I was receiving only an 'academic salary'. It was well known that such salaries in NYC paid just about one-half of the amount received by pathologists who worked in a hospital outside the large metropolitan area, and if one did not mind going a few hundred miles further away, the salaries could be even much higher. I did not mind this difference in income because, in my first years of practicing pathology, I wanted to try to pursue an academic career. Many of my colleagues, those with larger families or with previous financial obligations, moved out of the metropolitan area immediately after finishing the residency training. They took jobs in far-out locations. One went as far as Arizona, another to Arkansas, and another was in

Vermont, etc., and they received salaries that enabled them to buy a house without any delay, and with very light mortgage burden.

With time, I, too, had a growing family that required moving from an apartment into a house. A moonlighting position as director of a private laboratory was financially very effective: it required relatively little time, and it offered excellent remuneration. On two occasions, acting as director of a privately owned free-standing laboratory, I learned a few things about clinical laboratory business that were not at all covered during my residency training. *

One day, I received a phone call from John, a young medical lab technologist who had known me from the time of my residency training. After the usual introductory chit-chat, he asked me if I would be interested in taking the position of Director of Laboratory in a new private lab that was being financed and set up by his uncle. John would be the lab manager, but a licensed pathologist was needed for directorship and for handling cytology and tissue biopsies. He proceeded to outline the details of the entire undertaking: I would need to prepare the technical manuals for the clinical lab operation and as well for the quality assurance program, as required by the State Department of Health. The lab would be in a commercial building in a suburb, which, incidentally, was not too far from my home. Towards the end of our conversation, he quoted the monthly remuneration, which was more than satisfactory. The position would be quite stimulating - setting up a lab would require a lot of my time upfront,

---

* A free-standing medical laboratory usually performs general hematology, chemistry, bacteriology and serology testing but does not do blood compatibility (transfusion) testing. Free-standing labs also offer cytology and tissue biopsy services, for which they must employ a certified pathologist.

but it would also serve me well in maintaining my skills for running and controlling a clinical laboratory. Of course, I accepted the offer.

John's uncle requested my resume, and shortly thereafter, he interviewed me in a sumptuously furnished office, curiously located in an old, dilapidated building in a seedy part of the Bronx. During the interview, it became evident that John's uncle knew about me and my family a lot more than what was in my resume. He impressed me as a very shrewd businessman who researched every detail of my background. A couple of days later, John called and let me know that his uncle approved my position as director of the new lab. His uncle would also see to it that the lab receives plenty of work, that is, patients' tests from private medical clinics and from doctors' offices in NYC. I soon provided John with a list of equipment and supplies needed to run the lab, and I started to write the manuals of operation. After six weeks of intense preparatory work, the lab was completely set up and ready to start functioning. John hired several young medical technologists, the State inspected the new lab and issued a permit, and the lab was opened and began to work. I visited every day late in the afternoon, on the way home from my regular job, and everything was running smoothly, without any hitch.

One evening, about a month later, there was a knock on our house door. Standing outside in the dark was a young man, who I never saw before, and when I opened the door, he said:

"Hi! I am from the lab! I have your salary."

"Please, come in!"

Stepping into the foyer, the man reached into his pants pocket, pulled out a roll of bills, quickly counted out the monthly salary in hundreds, and handed it to me. I counted, found it correct, and said:

"Thank you! Now, where do I…" but he cut me off:

"Good night!" and he turned around, starting to leave. I quickly touched his elbow and repeated:

"Where do I sign? The receipt!"

Turning around, he looked at me for a second, then smiled and said: "Nah... nah... we trust you!"

"Well, thank you! Have a good night!"

That was an unusual way to pay a salary, but what did I know? New York was a big city, and I came from a very small place. John's uncle also struck me as being a little unusual, but everything else was normal. My salary was good, and it came on time. After working in that lab for three months, I began to feel uncomfortable: I was receiving a monthly salary of three thousand dollars, all in cash and without having to sign a receipt. On my next regular lab visit, just before leaving, I said to John:

"Hey, John, would it be possible to mail me the salary? I mean, a check! It would save the lab driver a whole trip to my house."

"Cash is better, doc! But, if that's how you want it, it's OK with us. We'll send you a check. Have a good night!"

"Good night!"

The following month, my salary check came promptly by mail. I deposited it and felt much better. I knew that my tax accountant liked it better when the income was received by check. The check, though, was from the "X... Hauling Company", with the address of the office where I was interviewed for the job. I began to think: John's uncle was the owner of a hauling company, but I had no idea what kind of hauling this company did. A friend of mine explained that 'hauling' usually referred to trucking of refuse, garbage, and he informed me of some other types of business that might be associated with hauling.

Then I understood why John's uncle took such pain in knowing everything about me and my background, including who my first cousin was, what his profession was, etc... I also remembered that the entire back wall of the uncle's office was decorated by a full-size color picture from a recent most popular movie, "The Godfather", showing the portrait of the whole family... I did not have to think much before deciding to resign from that job.

On my next visit to the lab, after finishing the work, I went to John's office and said:

"John, I have to tell you something important! I am sorry, but as of the end of this month, I will have to resign!" He looked at me in disbelief:

"But why? What do you mean? Everything's going so good!"

"Yeah, and I have been very happy working for you! But unfortunately, the boss at my hospital just told me that I can no longer keep an outside job."

"Well, OK, but you can't just leave us in a lurch! You first better find another pathologist who can replace you! And have him immediately submit his resume to my uncle! You know the address..."

"Of course, I'll find someone suitable as soon as I can."

It was easy! I had no trouble finding a young pathologist who was very happy to take my place. John and I parted on the friendliest of terms. This was the shortest moonlighting job I ever had.

Only then did I realize that anyone, just having enough money, can get a permit to own and run a medical facility, a lab, a clinic, or a pharmacy, just like a gas station or a bar, or any shop. I still don't know if there is any hope that someday, some governing body, before issuing a permit for operation of a medical facility, will be mindful of the fact that a business which deals with human health and human lives, and not with bricks and lumber, should be permitted to operate after a better scrutiny of its owner's source of finances and personnel.

Not long after that episode, I got another position of directorship, also in a free-standing private lab, and that moonlighting job lasted much longer. The offer for that new job came to me one day at work, while I was talking with a lab technologist in the hospital. His name was Jerry Parenti, he was about thirty years old, and he told me that he was getting tired of working for the hospital. Together with several of his friends, all of them lab technologists, he told me, he was about to start a jointly owned private medical lab. By pooling their savings, the technologists had already set up a corporation, and they only needed to find and hire a Director of Laboratory. Jerry's corporation was already negotiating to rent a space in a newly built suburban building and was planning to lease the furniture and all necessary lab equipment. The lab work would come from the offices of various doctors and clinics in NYC, places that his corporate partners knew from their current and prior jobs. My proposed salary would be three thousand dollars per month, apparently the going rate for directorship of a private lab. It sounded good: Jerry didn't have any support from an 'uncle', and I accepted the position.

From my previous work in a private lab, I already had copies of manuals for procedures and quality control, and I could easily adjust them to any newly leased equipment. The lab operation could start as soon as the furniture and equipment were installed and operational, and, of course, inspected and certified by the State. The lab location was again in a suburb, where I could conveniently stop by in the afternoon or evening on the way home from my hospital job. Jerry gave me a simple contract, typed on the letterhead of his corporation. Soon, I visited the rented premises, and I was impressed with the ample space and most modern equipment leased by the corporation. Very quickly, the State visited and certified the lab, and within a few days, the lab started receiving the work: lab tests and lots of cytology specimens (PAP smears). Within a month, the lab handled a very large volume of tests with the greatest efficiency. One could see that this was a well-organized business, run and managed by experienced technologists who owned it.

Obviously, Jerry and his friends had good connections with multiple clinics and doctors' offices in and around NYC, and it was clear from the workload that the corporation would earn an excellent income. For my part, there was quite a bit more work than I expected, especially with cytology slides, which I preferred to take home and do in the evenings on my own microscope. I did not mind doing the extra work, and the remuneration was very good. Five times a week, I stopped at the lab to check the quality control results and to pick up the cytology work. On weekends, I made longer visits to the lab to thoroughly check each specific testing area, and I found everything running "like a clockwork". At the end of each month, the lab corporation regularly mailed my check.

About eleven months after the lab started operating, during one of my evening visits, Jerry mentioned that the corporation might have a favorable offer to be taken over. The potential buyer only needed some time, to verify the work volume and the cash flow. A month later, Jerry let me know, that the lab received a very good cash offer, and he and his partners decided to sell. He asked whether I would be willing to continue serving as director with the future owner. I wanted to first meet the new owner, but since he was out of state, I spoke with him only by phone. He was a businessman who already hired a crew of technologists, and after a short discussion, we tentatively agreed on my continued position with the same salary.

Meanwhile, the sale of the lab occurred very quickly, so that one evening, about a week later, when I arrived at the lab, I met the new owner in person. He informed me that the new crew of technologists had visited the lab already a couple of days before the formal transfer of ownership, so that the new staff was familiar with all lab equipment and could continue to work without any disruption. I met most of the new staff, and it was a mixed group, including two experienced technologists. During the first week with the new owner, I checked the lab operation very rigorously and found it running just as smoothly as before.

One evening, at the end of the second week under the new owner, he called me into his little office to talk. He told me that over the last few days, the workload had begun to decrease. Nearly a quarter of the work volume shown on the books before he bought the lab, was no longer coming in. Some of the clinics and doctors' offices were not giving the lab messenger any work. When he approached those clinics and offices, he was told that they contracted with another lab. In the middle of the following week, I found that the owner dismissed more than half of the technologists. The lab received less than half of the usual workload, and I had to do very little cytology. The owner again called me into his office and told me that "something has gone very wrong". He showed me some letters that arrived during that week, addressed to the old corporate name of the lab, and all containing notices showing months of arrears in payments for leased equipment and furniture, and threatening to repossess everything if the payments were not received within the next five business days.

It turned out that during the last eleven months, only the first three or four months of leases had been paid for; thereafter, the payments never resumed, despite repeated requests and warnings. Some of the letters were also from companies that provided lab supplies and chemicals, and they also threatened to stop deliveries, unless they received past-due payments within a week. The owner tried to contact Jerry, but he was apparently out of town, and the other corporate partners were also unreachable. This well-run and successful lab, after having been sold for cash, turned out to be a scam! Jerry and his corporate friends made a handsome profit, both from a year of the lab's operation and from the cash sale, but then they somehow neglected to maintain the flow of work from doctors' offices and clinics. I went home and wrote a letter of resignation and, the following evening, handed it to the new owner. He accepted it, paid my salary for three weeks, and we parted with expressions of regret.

At about the same time, I discovered a problem with my last two paychecks from Jerry's corporation. The checks, one right after the other, were returned to me from my local bank, both stamped "insufficient funds".

When I inquired at my bank, the teller advised me to go to the bank where the checks were drawn and cash them right there. Jerry's corporation had an account at a large, nationally known bank (today still one of the largest in the country), let's call it the "Big Bank". The account was at a branch located in a rather desolate part of the Bronx. I went there, presented the checks to a teller, and she immediately sent me to see the branch manager. When he saw the checks, the manager looked at me and started talking very rapidly, as if he was in a great hurry:

"These corporate checks are good! They are perfectly OK! But just this moment, the corporate account has, as you can see it marked, insufficient funds. We believe that more funds for this corporate account are due to come in soon, very soon! You should wait just a few more days, or better, wait for one week! Then go and just re-deposit the checks at your bank, and it will be fine!"

He appeared to be a busy man, and I thanked him for his time and left. Yes, it had to be true: only three weeks after selling the lab, Jerry's corporation should still be receiving lots of late payments for the tests done during previous months…

A week later, when I went to cash the checks at my local bank, the teller immediately told me that once a check was stamped "insufficient funds", it was no longer acceptable, and it could be cashed only at the originating bank. I went back to that bank branch, and the busy manager gave me again the same story, claiming that "just this moment", the account had no funds to cover the checks. I began to see that the branch manager of the Big Bank worked hand in hand with Jerry and his friends, who directed him on how to handle their money. I felt that in such a case, it was better not to make a big fuss about it with the upper management of that bank. Instead, I kept trying to call Jerry, but his phone just rang and rang, without an answer.

I was holding in my hands two paychecks for a total of six thousand dollars, a nice sum in the mid-seventies. I decided to try cashing the checks in a different way. I opened a new personal savings account at the Big Bank, but in a nice branch, in Manhattan. There I deposited one of the two checks from Jerry's corporation, which was 3,000 dollars, and it was received without a fuss. The next day, I went to the same branch and withdrew 2,995 dollars in cash, leaving 5 dollars on the account. A few days later, I returned to deposit the second check from Jerry's corporation. This time, right upon seeing my check, the teller immediately asked me to see the branch manager. He received me in a friendly manner, and after the usual introduction, he looked at my check and handed it back to me, saying:

"Please, hold on to this. You know…, we have a problem with the first check you deposited. It appears, that this account has insufficient funds. Now, please, you should return to us the cash you have withdrawn from your account. Please, do it as soon as possible, will you?"

"Well, there should be really no problem with that check! It is from your bank, the "Big Bank", just from another branch! I am sure that you can settle the issue of insufficient funds with the manager of that branch! He should be able to make it good. After all, you both work for the same bank!"

"Yeah, but this is not as simple as you think!

"Well… I know that this corporate account is still receiving plenty of payments for its past services. The manager of that branch has told me so. There should be sufficient money to cover both of my checks. It is up to the manager of that branch to distribute the money where it belongs!"

"Well, will see… but for now, you should first return the cash—" but I cut him off:

"The cash has been spent! Please, do call your colleague, the manager at the other branch, to straighten the problem." I bid him goodbye and left.

I remained stuck with one bad check for 3,000 dollars, and I could console myself that I lost only one month's salary, not two. In summary, this moonlighting job gave me a rich experience in more than one way, and I had no regrets. It was very satisfactory to be able to set up an entire clinical lab for a second time, control the quality of testing, and perform all the other duties of a lab director for a whole year. It was an experience that would serve me well in the future. It also helped to lighten the mortgage load on our house.

About two months after resigning from that lab, I finally managed to catch Jerry on the phone. He gave me a long and sad story, which I listened to with great interest. He had suffered "a great misfortune" and was "completely devastated" so that he had to go away for several weeks to rest at his cousin's house in New Jersey. Right after the sale of the lab, he said, he went to the bank to deposit the money, but on the way there, he ran into a terrible traffic jam. Two tenements were burning, and the fire trucks blocked several streets. He parked his Cadillac and went to have a sandwich in a little bar. About half an hour later, when he returned to the car, the lock on the trunk was broken, and his bag with all the cash and corporate books were stolen. He and his partners were "left with nothing" and they did not even have enough money to cover some debts from the time they started the corporation. Finally, he said, he was very sorry that there was nothing left to cover my last two checks. He ended the whole soap story, sadly declaring:

"You know, I'll have to get out of town and take a job! I hope to get one in Las Vegas." I said goodbye and wished him better luck in Vegas. He sounded so desperate, as if getting a job and working was going to be the worst calamity in his life.

During the following several months, the Big Bank started going after me. I kept receiving letters requesting a return of the money that I cashed out of my savings account. Soon after that, I moved out of town and started a new job, quite far from NYC, and I ignored the letters from the bank.

A couple of months later, after I was well settled in my new job, my small local bank sent me a notice that my personal account has been blocked due to an "unpaid debit" at the Big Bank. As a result, all payments due from my account were stopped, and this was quite embarrassing. Well, I learned that the Big Bank had long arms and played rough. I had to urgently engage a local attorney, who quickly documented I was not at fault. My local bank account was unblocked within two days.

Two years after the episode with Jerry's corporate lab, there was a little sequel. I received a letter from a bankruptcy court in NYC, inquiring whether I had any claims regarding Jerry's lab corporation. Somehow, a copy of the allegedly stolen corporate books was found, and since my name was on the payroll, the court dutifully traced me down to my new location. I was still in possession of the one bad check for 3,000 dollars, kept as a souvenir. I chose not to make any claim nor to respond to the inquiry. I did not wish to have any further connection with that lab corporation.

Several years passed by, and the unsavory episode with Jerry became a vague memory, but then, a curious coincidence made me remember him. I had a good friend, a neighbor around the corner from our house. His name was Angelo, and he worked as for a local business. He and his wife, Maria, had gone on a short visit to NYC to celebrate their 25th anniversary, and while there, Angelo went to the 49th Street diamond district to do a little shopping. He purchased a diamond ring as an engagement present for his son's fiancée. After Angelo and Maria returned home, they invited Miriam and me to join them for an evening with espresso and a glass of wine. While we chatted, Angelo pulled out of his pocket a little box and showed us the diamond he bought. As he held the ring high up in the air, it sparkled, and we admired it. The diamond was quite large, and I asked if he had it checked for quality. Angelo was a savvy guy, and he just smiled. He knew very well how important it was that a gem has a good cut and color, and purity. Then he joked, saying that buying a diamond does not take as long as buying a house, but it does take more time than buying a pair of pants. When I looked at the diamond, it shone with all colors: it was just beautiful. Angelo, meanwhile, pulled out a piece of paper and showed us that he received an appraiser's warranty for the gem. It was a fancy folded card that looked almost like someone's university diploma, a certificate guaranteeing the gem's purity, size, etc. My eye fell on the well-practiced, completely illegible signature of the appraiser, and below it, in ornate, large gold letters, the printed name: JERRY PARENTI. I felt a slow rise of blood in my head. Turning to Angelo, I just said:

"What a fancy signature! Must be an old man!"

"Oh, no! He was middle-aged and a smart dresser, very professional."

"Tall, dark, and quite handsome!" added Maria.

"Well, you bought a gorgeous diamond!" and I handed the certificate back to Angelo. While he was putting the diamond ring into its box, I wondered if it was possible that it was the same Jerry Parenti I knew from the lab. The description of his appearance seemed to fit…

The rest of the evening, the four of us talked happily, and we came to the idea of taking a little vacation from the dreary winter to join for a short retreat on a Caribbean island. And all the while, in the back of my mind, I kept remembering Jerry. It was entirely possible that a few people share the same first and last name. All the same, I had a distinct feeling that this was Jerry, the lab technologist I knew from before. I thought, *Jerry would be perfectly capable of returning from Las Vegas with a diploma of an appraiser of precious stones.*

About two years later, Angelo told me that the marriage of his son unfortunately ended in a divorce after only one year. If I were superstitious, I would believe that it was on account of the diamond ring, because anything Jerry touched, would have a jinx on it.

Chapter 8
Teaching and Research

When I started my training in pathology, I had a real interest in teaching and research, and I thought of a possible career in academic medicine. However, I also wanted to practice pathology and put to full use my skills and knowledge how to make a proper, correct diagnosis. I hoped that practicing in an academic center would give me an opportunity to see what a career devoted to teaching and research would entail.

I grew up in old Europe, where being a university professor and teaching at a medical school, at least in the first half of the twentieth century, was an honorable position that was valued, respected, and well-rewarded. In my position at a medical school in NYC, I spent eight years practicing diagnostic pathology, while also teaching and doing research, and I found that in the second half of twentieth century, it was still a nice position, but the conditions about it have changed in a way that I did not expect.

The teaching part of my job was twofold. During the school semester, I was assigned to give several lectures and multiple lab sessions with medical students, but throughout the entire year I did daily teaching of residents in pathology. Training of the residents was done by means of diagnostic sign-out conferences and performing jointly with residents the frozen sections with rapid diagnosis. Working with residents was easy: they were eager to learn the skills of their future profession. Due to the chronic shortage of physicians from US medical schools, most residents in my program came from other countries: Bolivia, China, Germany, India, Iran, Korea, Philippines,

Yugoslavia, etc. Managing the residency training program provided some interesting moments.

In my first year of teaching at the medical school I encountered a resident from Iran, who stood out, being always neatly dressed and well groomed, apparently coming from an affluent family. I took notice of him after he was reported exhibiting a peculiar stunt that did not go well with his colleagues. Whenever he was asked to do a service chore that he did not like, he pretended not to understand English sufficiently enough to grasp what was required. As he repeatedly pulled the same trick with other residents, I began to hear more and more complaints about him. However, when talking with me, his command of English appeared quite adequate. After this wise guy did his trick one time too many, the Chief Resident came to me and asked for a formal intervention.

I called the resident into my office and made it clear that his refusal to do certain chores was unacceptable and that he better stop feigning poor understanding of English. With me, he took a different tack. Speaking with a fair command of English, he proceeded to tell me:

"I am guest in your country, and, you know… guest must receive courtesy! They should speak to me in Farsi. Then I will know what they want."

"Are you saying, we should learn to speak Farsi?"

"Yes, it is good courtesy!"

This was so brazen, that I only told him not to worry, the problem would be taken care of. I analyzed the record of his performance and found that we had a series of complaints about him, and nothing positive. He knew exactly what he was doing. It did not matter whether he was a rich, arrogant brat or whether he had just a quirky personality, but he had to be stopped. I sent the case to the senior council of the department, questioning the possibility of having him dismissed from the program. At their next meeting, the council made a unanimous decision to have the resident summarily fired if he were to commit another infraction. That did not take long, and I had my very first experience of having someone fired from his job. Not a pleasant task, but it had to be done.

We also had a resident who was an especially nice fellow, well-liked by everyone. He was reliable, diligent and courteous, and he never missed a day's work. Except, one day, in his third year of residency, he did not show up for work. This was most unusual, and the Chief Resident covered up for him without reporting it. The following day, I was informed that our good resident failed to appear at work for a second day, and without any notice or excuse. Several phone calls to his home were not answered. The Chief Resident was frustrated, and he finally came to me and said:

"I don't understand it! For him, this is completely out of character!"

I asked our departmental secretary to keep trying to call the resident's home. Sooner or later, someone would have to answer the phone. At the end of the day, the secretary came to my office and reported that even after multiple attempts, no one ever answered the listed phone number. The next morning, the same secretary ran into my office, all excited, with a newspaper in hand. She handed me the paper, saying:

"Dr. Yellinek, please see here! This is about our missing resident!" Below is a summary of the news article.

Our resident was described as a young physician, a bachelor, and an immigrant from Bolivia with no known family in US. He lived in a sublet room, in the apartment that belonged to a middle-aged lady from his country. His landlady was unattached, and she owned a butcher shop in the vicinity of the apartment. The physician and the landlady had been romantically involved. About two years into this relationship, the physician started seeing another younger woman. When the landlady discovered that liaison, she became very upset and angry. For several nights, she suffered and wasn't able to fall asleep. One night, angry and desperate, she went to her kitchen, took a butcher knife, and while her tenant was sleeping, she quietly entered his room. For a while, she stood over him and watched him sleeping. Suddenly, she felt a great surge of anger, uncovered him, and stabbed him in the abdomen. When she saw the blood gushing from his belly, she ran to the phone and called an ambulance. Unfortunately, by the time help arrived, he had bled to death. When the police arrived, the landlady broke down, started crying, and then admitted what happened. The man was pronounced dead, and the landlady was arrested…

There was one more unusual resident story, and it's about a resident who secretly dated a secretary in our office. Working in the same department, both managed for a very long time to keep their relationship under cover. The secretary was in her mid-twenties, a tall, well-built girl with a pretty face, blue eyes, and light brown hair. She was an only child and lived with her parents in New Jersey. The resident, in his early thirties, handsome, with black hair and dark eyes, was always polite and courteous and otherwise mostly quiet. He eventually met the girl's parents, and the two of them were regularly going out on weekends and some evenings. After nearly two years of steady courtship, right after he was promoted to Chief Resident, the two of them got engaged. It was the month of April, and the secretary one day appeared in the office with a ring on her hand, and finally let the news of the engagement spread through the whole pathology department. Congratulations were given and received. The resident was about to graduate from our training program at the end of June of that year, and the couple was planning for an August wedding, after the resident obtained a steady job.

Fourth of July was the usual long weekend, and everyone was off. When I came back to work on the morning after the holiday, I found our secretary in obvious distress. Her eyes and face were all red from crying, and I invited her into my office to see if I could do anything to help. She said that over the long weekend, she was to meet her fiancé at her girlfriend's apartment in the City, and they were to spend some time together, but for the first time ever, inexplicably, her fiancé did not show up. Finally, she said:

"He just vanished, like… disappeared from the Earth!"

"What do you mean?"

"We could not find him anywhere…" and she slowly explained to me what happened. Her girlfriend, who usually let the couple use her apartment when they wanted some privacy, claimed that she had not seen the fiancé after their last mutual visit, about one week earlier. When our secretary rang the home telephone number of the fiancé, there was a message saying: "This number has been discontinued." She finally took a long subway ride to a very distant part of Brooklyn and went to his apartment. Ringing at his apartment, there was no answer to the door. The building janitor said that the apartment was vacated on June 29th and would be soon ready for rental. The janitor did not receive any forwarding address…

It took more than one week before the mystery of the vanished young pathologist was resolved. The parents of our hapless secretary were able to track him down through a private agency, partly with the help of the immigration service. He was in a town not far from the Canadian border, where he just accepted a job as an assistant pathologist in the local hospital. His wife, with two children, had just recently arrived from Korea and joined him at his new location.

* * *

Teaching the medical students was divided into three parts: lectures to a large class of about 200, lab sessions with groups of about 35, and occasional tutoring of individual students. The experience with the students also turned out to be educational for me. In my first year, I was assigned to give only a few lectures, and it was an activity that I really enjoyed. I was given a fair latitude in how to design the lectures. One of the assigned topics was "The Pathology of Malnutrition", which was well covered in the students' textbook under the title "Vitamin Deficiencies." Instead of that, I chose to give a talk about the ills of obesity, a topic that was in those years not much covered in the textbook, and I observed that it was in the surrounding environment much more prevalent than malnutrition.

For the student lab sessions, I had to prepare materials covering a review of the entire pathology course by demonstrating preserved pathologic tissue samples and as well by projecting microscopic images of pathologic changes, followed by a discussion. A part of the session was also devoted to probing the students' knowledge with pertinent questions. If any student showed very poor knowledge, this had to be reported to a senior professor in charge of student education. Most students were very good or satisfactory, but as it happens in every large class, there were always a few individuals who displayed a surprising level of ignorance and disinterest in the subject of pathology.

At the regular monthly meetings of our department, it came out that those deficient students ought to be tutored on a one-to-one basis, and we had to schedule and conduct special tutoring sessions. The rationale for tutoring was that our department had a policy that no student should ever fail to graduate on account of failing in pathology. I never understood that sort of attitude. I approached teaching with the simple idea that a student who does not pass the exam in any subject should not get an MD degree. Anyway, I tutored several students, and most improved and passed the exam, but on two occasions, my tutoring was all in vain, and the student simply would not bother to make an effort to learn pathology. When I raised this issue with the professor in charge of student education, he just shrugged and said: "Oh, don't worry! It will all work out! The weak ones graduate and then find a niche in Public Health, where they don't practice with patients. Eventually, they'll add to their MD an MPH degree (Master of Public Health) and will end up in management and politics, where they can't do any harm to a patient!"

And indeed, in the subsequent years, I noticed an ever-increasing number of MDs with a degree of MPH, though many of them did practice with patients.

Our medical school participated in an effort to alleviate the national shortage of physicians, and to that end, it introduced a fast-track curriculum. The students would graduate from medical school in three years instead of the usual four. That three-year curriculum squeezed into each year an additional summer semester, and it was quite demanding, both for the students and for the teaching staff. The program generated an immediate large influx of money to the school, coming from the federal government. It was a well-deserved award for faster production of physicians. An interesting phenomenon occurred three years later when, at the end of the school year, there were two separate classes of graduating MDs, though one class graduated two months later than the other. Several years later, the stressful three-year program was terminated, and the school switched back to the normal four-year curriculum. Three years down the road, that change resulted in a year without any graduation.

With time, I was getting assigned an increasing load of student lectures. Nearly half of all lectures and all lab sessions for students were assigned to the junior staff in our department, and relatively few lectures were given by senior professors. About half of all lectures were assigned to the visiting clinicians, the MDs who practiced at our hospital and were willing to volunteer as lecturers. In return, the school gave them the title of "Clinical Assistant Professor," a useful addition to the letterhead and the shingle at the office.

The fact that most lectures were relegated to clinicians and to the junior staff made me feel that student lectures were not of foremost importance. The mere act of teaching was neither much valued, nor was it well rewarded. This was true not only in pathology but also in other basic medical courses, such as anatomy, physiology, microbiology, etc., which were not taught by MDs, but by PhDs, whose main interest was in their research and not in teaching. The lesson I learned about teaching at the medical school was that a professor was valued and well rewarded not for teaching, but only for research, which provided rich grants with ample funding.

The pathology course was taught for two full semesters, and the medical students received only one semester of anatomy. In that single semester of anatomy, the students would learn the mere basics about the abdomen, chest and part of the head and nervous system. There was no time to learn any anatomy of the extremities, bones, joints, eyes, ears, or other small organs. When I quizzed the students about the number of menisci in the knee joint, their answers were guesses, ranging from "one" to "four". One of the staff clinicians explained to me that only a specialist, in this case, an orthopedic surgeon, needed to know the anatomy of the bones, joints and extremities. Knowing the anatomy of the eye would be needed only by an ophthalmologist. On the other hand, the students were taught the fine ultrastructure of inner cell components that could be seen only with an electron microscope and would be useful only to someone who wanted to become a professional researcher. I never understood how a physician can practice quality medicine without knowing the complete anatomy of the human body.

I reflected on my own medical education, which included five semesters of pathology and four semesters of anatomy, so that as an MD, I would know and understand the function of all parts of the human body. Clearly, I attended an antiquated medical school, where all professors were MDs, except the one PhD in biochemistry, and all were experts in their subject. The memory of my school began to feel like a fable from a distant planet in the past century. The current system of medical education is geared to produce specialists, where a neurologist needs to know the nervous system, and an ear, nose, and throat specialist must know only about those three little organs, as if they were neither connected nor dependent on the rest of the human body.

Over the years, my joy in giving lectures and holding student labs was gradually ebbing away. It was still pleasing to give a lecture and see that a large class was mostly paying attention, with only very few chatting, or doing some private business, or falling asleep. (Cell phones and Internet did not exist!) My only fulfillment from teaching came from a few individual students, who in lab sessions actively showed an interest and appreciation for learning.

*   *   *

The importance of research at the medical school became known to me only after I spent some time around the large group of researchers in our department. The research lab was richly appointed, and all equipment was provided by funds from various grants. While doing my own little research in that lab, I had the opportunity to see how the big academic research was conducted, how it functioned, and how it was possible to stretch it into a whole life career.

Most of the research was done by teams of three, four, or more people, where every member had a well-defined role. One of the crucial tasks of the team was to write a successful application for funding, the "grant application," usually addressed to NIH or a similar body. The application had to contain two main points: 1. describe the intended goal of the research, and 2. document and explain the importance of the expected results of that research. At least one team member had to have a special talent to write a good, "strong" grant application, meaning that the grant would not only be approved, but it would be well funded. A poorly written application might be "approved," but with too little or no funding… Next, I learned that writing a "strong" grant application usually took the same amount of time as the remaining part of the research that would be done after the grant was approved! The reason was that one had to complete a large part of a given research project and see at least some results before being able to document the importance of the project, and thereby write a "strong" grant application.

The largest research grant was held by the Chairman of the Department. Several senior members of the research group also held individual grants that provided funding of variable sizes. Consequently, our large research group of MDs and PhDs had several teams, each one doing research on a different subject. Occasionally, when a grant application was not funded, the researcher and his team would be temporarily "carried," that is, had their salaries supported by the Chairman's grant.

From the talk among researchers, it was easy to tell when the deadline for an important grant application was approaching. There was a certain sense of tension, mixed with anxiety, silently wafting in the air around the involved team members. Later, when the team received a favorable approval, with the expected "full funding," there would be a perceptible buzz throughout the entire research lab, and it would be followed by a small celebration. A little party with refreshments would be organized in one of the meeting rooms, and all members of the department would be invited. Those happy parties usually began at the end of a workday and lasted well into the evening.

How did the grant applications get approved, and who gave the approval? In general, it was known that some of the nationally prominent scientists and researchers, many of them grant receivers themselves, were invited by NIH and similar agencies to sit on their committees and evaluate grant applications. It was no secret that at least two of the senior members of our department sat on such committees. Beyond that, the process of approving and funding the grant applications remained for me a mystery.

The disposition of the funds from research grants was not at all a secret. All funds were deposited and kept in the bank account of the medical school. Monies were disbursed only upon a specific request made by the principal grant holder. When money was spent on supplies or equipment, the medical school would get an equal amount of money for its administrative services. However, when research funds were used toward salaries, the medical school would receive two dollars for every one dollar spent for a salary. The math of it was very simple: more than half of all grant money was used by the school for its own needs, while the research itself consumed the remaining part. This type of fiscal arrangement with grant monies was apparently customary throughout the academic world, and it is one of the few arrangements that appears to have remained unchanged over many years. I felt that it would not be objectionable if the medical school took even two-thirds of all grant money for its services, for the school was in the business of "producing" new physicians. The rationale is that our country needs many more MDs, and many physicians continue to be hired from abroad.

When I first started to do research, at the time of residency training, I was not aware that all research was divided into two main types: "basic science research" and "clinical research". While clinical research seeks findings that are directly applicable to patient care, basic science research is conducted with a deeper purpose, where the results and findings may be very important sometime in the future. My research on amyloid was in the realm of "basic science". The pathologists and doctoral scientists who conducted research in our department were, with few exceptions, almost exclusively interested in making discoveries in basic science.

The basic science findings provide "building blocks," or foundations, that might prove to be useful later. The idea is that a basic foundational finding would give rise to further research in the same direction and would eventually add new findings to form another building block, on top of which one could add yet more findings, presenting a new, higher foundation, until someday, all these basic building blocks could be amalgamated into a great, valuable discovery… On some occasions, great discoveries do happen in this manner, but most of those basic "building blocks" remain forever in the process of further buildup, without ever being completed or used for any purpose. The process reminds me of Escher's paintings of staircases that lead high up, and end with the top stair perched in the air - without a landing.

Basic science research continuously produces new substrates, from which one may continue further research… The results of basic research usually answer one specific question, and along with it, they open a whole series of new questions that could be solved only by doing more research… In this manner, one has at hand a mechanism to perpetuate and continue research, literally "ad infinitum", without an end. That should explain how and why so many academic professionals are able to use basic science research to build themselves a whole life career.

One well-known motto among researchers is: "Publish or perish!" A researcher who does not publish some new findings or cannot obtain a grant for his research would better switch to another profession. There was (and still is) in the research community a tremendous pressure to publish as many papers as possible. An average researcher's success and career trajectory is measured mainly by the number of published papers and, only in rare cases, by an extraordinary discovery. To earn recognition, a researcher must be able to publish at least some of the papers in the more prestigious "reviewed journals". With all this pressure to publish, there should be no surprise that the research community harbors, along with a true zeal for discovery, also a great deal of competition, jealousy, outright enmity, in-fighting, and sometimes pitiably, plagiarized, false or invented data.

Those who follow medical literature will notice that there are hundreds of medical and biological journals that publish thousands of papers every month, but only about two to three percent show findings of some value. The other 97 percent serve as page fillers and carry little or no significance. This is not surprising when one remembers that the world has tens of thousands of researchers, and each year, only a handful make a great discovery. There is a reason why such a huge quantity of published papers shows only a small number of truly valuable results. The reason becomes at least partly evident when one reads the statistics on scientific discoveries, which reveal that the vast majority of important, valuable discoveries are made by people in their twenties, much less in their thirties, and only very exceptionally by people older than forty. Despite such statistics, most of the large research grants in the academic world continue to be awarded to senior scientists who are in their forties, fifties and sixties. Those are the life-career researchers who know how to continuously obtain grants with ample funding, while employing and using young, talented people to do their research.

Reading the daily press, one can also find reports about research papers published, sometime in reputable journals, showing data that are later proven false and are then retracted. This phenomenon is attributed to the enormous pressure to publish and to obtain more grant money. In some cases, the findings of false data are revealed by other scientists, who, while trying to repeat a published finding, are unable to reproduce the original results.

There has been lately an ever-increasing number of falsified data in scientific publications, discovered with the aid of AI. At the same time, there have been many embarrassing retractions of papers coming from some well-known universities and from reputable journals.

Back in the sixties, there used to be a small publication called "Journal of Irreproducible Results," that was both satirical and humorous. It came from a little country abroad, and it regularly addressed the issues of the quality of research or the lack of it. That journal, with its appropriately comical title, mocked the charlatanism, skullduggery, and falsifications that every now and then emanated from the people engaged in research. Reading that journal, one could see that the research community is made up of people who were no different from any other human group: both the good and the bad are represented.

After having published three papers of basic research, my preference turned to the clinical research projects. Then I found that in the seventies, clinical research was treated by the academic community as if it were of lesser value. Such treatment left an impression that only basic science research was an all-important, "high-class" endeavor.

The clinical research was treated as if it was inferior and unimportant. At that time, if one wanted to publish a paper about clinical research, for example, a description of a rare and unusual form of a disease, to help make a correct diagnosis, most medical journals would not accept it for publication. The editors of those journals displayed an attitude, preferring to publish only content of basic science research. Those who wanted to publish clinical research had to cope with that frivolous attitude.

On a personal level, when I tried to publish papers about diseases of practical interest, I often had a hard time getting my work accepted for publication. A perfectly useful clinical paper would be rejected by several journals, before it would be finally accepted. Later, in the eighties and nineties, the editorial attitude slowly changed, and clinical research began to be regularly accepted and published.

My clinical research was mostly involved with tumors and cancer, but here follows an example that was very different. One of our urologists designed a clinical research project with the objective of testing whether fertility in males could be re-established after vasectomy, and if it could be regulated by using a valve implant. The urologist found a fair number of volunteers willing to participate, mostly younger and middle-aged men. Working with an engineer, the urologist designed an implant composed of a small silver tube with a valve in it. By means of vasectomy, the implant could be inserted between two ends of a severed vas (sperm duct). The valve had a tiny handle that could be reached through the skin and thereby turned on and off at will.

One year following the bilateral implants of the tubes, all participants remained sterile, without evidence of any sperm flow, despite the valves being in a fully open position. The silver tubes were then surgically removed, and the sperm ducts were surgically reconnected. The tissue ends of silver tubes were pathologically examined, and I found that they were completely overgrown and blocked by massive growth of scar tissue. Six months after the sperm ducts were re-connected, there was still no evidence of sperm flow in any of the volunteers. In the next phase of the project, we received biopsies of the area where the sperm ducts were re-connected, and again, we found blockage by massive formation of scar tissue. The scaring was caused by the sperm cells, which are known to be severely allergenic when they come in contact with any tissue cells other than the intact inner lining of the sperm duct. In conclusion, this little project revealed that a vasectomy cannot be reversed, and that fertility cannot be regained, nor could it be regulated by a valve implant.

My involvement in research comprised only a small fraction of my career. It was a side activity that was completely voluntary, done for pleasure, and to satisfy a curiosity. As soon as I fully realized that findings in basic science produced only "building blocks" with a potential value in the future, my interest in that type of research waned. After going through the entire medical school and four years of residency training, a physician who then did just basic research, would be wasting all his practical medical knowledge. The fiercely competitive race for funding and the "grantsmanship" practiced by the career researchers was not to my taste. I felt it was better to continue with clinical research which yields practical results, and where one did not have to constantly write applications for funding. The nicest thing about clinical research is that it requires only some personal time and virtually no funds. I would remain in academic medicine only long enough to be qualified for directorship in a hospital with a strong oncology department, where I could practice diagnostic pathology.

Several of my friends and colleagues, who spent their entire careers doing basic research at medical schools, were dedicated and hard-driving individuals, who sincerely believed in their work, and I admired them. A few years ago, in retirement, I met with one of my colleagues who spent his entire career doing research for a chemical company. He was proud to have 50 patents recorded to his name (his company had regularly patented his work every six to eight months). Although all those patents did not produce a single marketable product, he felt happy and fulfilled with his achievements, which some day may yet become a basic building block for a great discovery.

Basic science research reminds me of the concept of "infinity," that beautiful sign made of a circle twisted into a figure 8. When I think of infinity, I don't mean a movement in a circle, repeating the same path and reaching nowhere but back onto itself. I mean, infinity as a simple straight line, reaching out into space, without an end… Or it represents the entire cosmic space, with its four dimensions. The concept of infinity is also present in Nature, the biosphere, the fauna and flora, within all its live creatures, with an inexhaustible number of natural laws and phenomena, many of which are yet to be discovered. At the same time, the mind of a single human being contains an infinite repository of thoughts and beliefs, straight or convoluted, logical or false, without an end. So, there is much more research to be done about the human mind, its brilliance, and its failings. I never understood, how is it possible, that the human mind can believe in ideas, subjects or objects which cannot be detected by any conscious human sense? That also, certainly requires more research.

Chapter 9

My Immediate Boss

Dr. Morton Braun, the Chief of Surgical Pathology at the main hospital of the medical school, was the immediate boss to Harry and me. I worked under Dr. Braun for full eight years, and he taught me several interesting concepts, procedures, and novelties in pathology. During those years, he also gave me lasting memories that deserve a separate chapter.

I first met Dr. Braun during the interview for the job when the Chairman of the Department introduced me and asked him to take me on a tour of the department. At first impression, Dr. Braun appeared somewhat intimidating: a middle-aged man of medium height with a large chest and a big, balding head, a tanned face, and a booming baritone voice. While taking me around the offices and work areas of the department, he walked briskly and with a swagger, and he spoke with the vigor and conviction fitting an owner of the hospital. I had to try hard to keep up with his pace. Using a few words, he explained that most of the time, he was involved with cancer research, and he needed help only for routine diagnostic services in surgical pathology and cytology. Then he introduced me to his assistant, Dr. Harry Knob, and a minute later, Dr. Braun looked at his watch, and then at me, and abruptly declared:

"Well... you will get your answer from the Chairman of the Department!", so I understood that the interview was over. As I thanked him for his time, it felt certain that it was Dr. Braun who would decide on that answer.

Dr. Braun was a full professor at the medical school, and he had been in the position of Chief of Surgical Pathology for many years, from a time way before the current Chairman of the Department with his team of a dozen researchers came over from another institution. On my first morning at work, Dr. Braun indicated that Harry and I would share all the work in diagnostic service, and he himself would get involved only if Harry and I needed assistance with a problem in making a diagnosis, or if one of us was absent. He pointed out dryly that my other duties, regarding management and training of residents and taking charge of the histology laboratory, were outlined in my contract. He showed no interest in those areas of my work.

An early riser, Dr. Braun was every morning the first to come in to work, and he would be sitting at his desk way before the arrival of office secretaries. To avoid the heavy rush-hour traffic from the suburb where he lived, Dr. Braun would leave home every morning at 5 am and be at work before 6. He would leave the office and drive home at 2 pm. Several times in my first week at work, I arrived at 7 am, an hour earlier than required, and found Dr. Braun already working in his office, reading or writing some notes. He had a small special research grant and maintained his own research laboratory with a single technologist, Frank. When I first met Frank, who wore a half-length lab coat and carried a tray with coffee, I thought, he was Dr. Braun's personal valet. Later, I found that Frank was not at all a certified technologist, but a loyal and devoted clerk, a "gofer," who did any chore ordered by the boss, including lab work, for which he was "trained on the job".

Dr. Braun's major interest was in cancer research, particularly cancer of the breast. By the time I started working for him, he had already published scores of papers on that subject. He discovered three distinct types of cellular reaction in lymph nodes draining breast cancer and developed a theory, claiming that one of those cell reactions signified a good cancer prognosis, whereas patients who had either of the remaining two reactions had a poor prognosis and would succumb to cancer. Dr. Braun also invented a new classification of breast cancer cells, a cell grading system that was different from that found in the textbooks of pathology. Every diagnostic report of breast cancer in our department had to indicate in a footnote Dr. Braun's cell grade and the type of lymph gland reaction if the glands were available.

The footnote was written in form of a number/letter code, which would serve for statistics in Dr. Braun's research. To function in the department, I had to immediately learn to recognize Dr. Braun's cell grades, types of lymph gland reactions, and their codes.

I found Dr. Braun's definition of lymph gland reactions hard to follow, because very often, not all glands showed the same type of reaction… The grade of cancer cells was also hard to choose, as each cell grade was poorly defined. Finally, I asked Harry, who had been using those codes for several years, what was the best way to learn and apply Dr. Braun's definitions. Upon hearing my question, Harry made an enigmatic face and quietly looked at me for a few seconds, then just shrugged and said:

"Just do it! Do it as you best can! And look… don't worry about it! The surgeons, anyway, don't have any use for these codes, except, perhaps Dr. Larimer, who is a personal friend of Dr. Braun. The rest of the clinicians read only the diagnosis and don't pay any attention to those codes!" That was not the answer to my question, but nevertheless, it was of some help. I followed Harry's advice and began to add below each breast cancer diagnosis a footnote with the required codes, just trying to "do my best". I could only hope it was done the right way.

Sometime in my second week at work, Dr. Braun appeared in a very benevolent mood and offered me to join him in his research. He said I could apply the technique of electron microscopy to enlarge on his theory of the prognostic value of lymph gland reactions to cancer. I was very happy and felt honored by his offer. Dr. Braun went on to explain that he wanted me to study and confirm by electron microscopy the three distinct reactions in lymph glands draining breast cancer. He asked me to start immediately collecting and preserving lymph gland tissue from breast cancer patients. This was not hard: we had at least six to seven breast cancer surgeries per week, and the special chemicals for tissue preservation were readily available in the electron microscopy lab. Meanwhile, I still had to learn to better distinguish those three patterns of reaction with the light microscope that I used in my daily diagnostic work.

One morning, as I walked in to greet Dr. Braun in his office, he said he wanted to introduce me to a new procedure called "fine needle aspiration" of tumors. This new method of quick cytologic assessment of tumors, prior to surgery, was developed in Sweden, and, at that time, was not yet widely practiced in the US. Dr. Braun learned it only recently while he was on a sabbatical leave, doing research in Stockholm. He was applying this procedure to all patients of Dr. Larimer admitted to the hospital for surgery on a breast tumor.

A thin gauge needle mounted on a syringe was used to penetrate the tumor and aspirate a few drops of tissue, which would then be expelled onto a glass slide and spread into a thin cellular smear. The smear was rapidly stained, and the spread of individual cells was immediately examined under the microscope. In most cases, one could quickly determine whether the tumor contained cancer cells or not. If the aspirated cells were definitely diagnostic of cancer, the surgeon could do his procedure much faster by avoiding a delay of about half an hour, while waiting for a diagnosis made by a "frozen section" of the tumor biopsy.

For several months, I followed Dr. Braun on his morning rounds and assisted with fine needle aspirations. I was staining the cell smears and learning how to make a diagnosis by using a simple new rapid stain. On some occasions, Dr. Braun encouraged me to perform the needle aspiration by myself, and I had to struggle to do it with a steady hand and hide from the patient the fact that it was one of my first attempts.

After a couple of months of working alongside Dr. Braun, he declared he was confident I could do the procedure all by myself. To reassure me, he said if I needed help with the diagnosis, he would be glad to come and give me assistance. Meanwhile, he would have more time for his research. The following day, Dr. Braun introduced me to his friend, Dr. Herbert Larimer, a highly respected surgeon who did exclusively breast surgery and had a large private office located near the hospital. He alone admitted to the hospital about two-thirds of all patients with a breast tumor, and I would have to do fine needle aspiration on all his patients.

When I asked Harry why he did not do needle aspirations of breast tumors, he said:

"Yeah, I was offered to learn it, but I declined. You know, I am not interested in doing research. I prefer to make a rapid diagnosis on a frozen section of a solid piece of tissue, rather than by looking at a smear with a few cells."

"But Harry, this is not research! It's a new way of making a quick cytologic diagnosis. It saves time in surgery!"

"Yes, but it's not a nationally accepted and approved procedure. I know they do it in Sweden, but here in US, it's still experimental." Harry was right, but within a year, the procedure became an accepted standard in the US.

I was glad to learn a new skill, but I also had a new chore. Dr. Braun usually had breakfast around 6:30 am in the doctor's lounge, together with Dr. Larimer, who gave him a list with clinical information, including mammogram findings on all his patients scheduled for breast surgery on that day.

Every morning, by 8 am, I appeared in Dr. Braun's office, and he handed me the list of patients on who I was to do a fine needle aspiration. The findings had to be reported to Dr. Larimer before he started surgery.

Over the next several years, I got to know Dr. Braun quite well. He was married, had two teenage children, and according to Harry, he was quite wealthy, that is, as Harry put it: "…his wife inherited a fortune from her family". I had no idea where and through what channels did Harry get all this information. I noticed that there were times when Dr. Braun was relaxed, even mellow, and had a really good day, but there were also days, when I could tell that he was, for whatever reason, tense like a gun that could go off any second. When he was in a good mood, he would sometimes read to me a poem or a limerick that he'd just composed early that same morning. This was not a surprise, as Harry had already alerted me that our boss had a knack for writing poetry. Among the numerous pathology books on his shelf, I spotted a volume of poems by Walt Whitman, which may have inspired him for poetry. On the top shelf, Dr. Braun also had row of books with his name on the cover. One day, he reached for one of those books and handed it to me, saying:

"This is yours!"

Curious and excited, I thanked him and took the book home. It was a short book with the title "General Pathology" that he wrote together with another pathologist. I read it in one evening.

On the days when Dr. Braun was tense, his mood was betrayed by ticks, either twitching of eyelids or taking several rapid inhaling breaths. He had a strong personality, and I quickly realized that it was best to stay on his good side. From many of his remarks, one could see that in most matters he was a rigid conservative. After we worked together for over a year, he felt free to express his opinions about the other members of the medical staff. Talking about people who he did not hold in high esteem, Dr. Braun used to simply refer to them as "those clowns". The tone with which he pronounced the word "clowns" would let you know exactly how he felt about them. I tried hard not to become one of "those", but as time went by, I am sure that I managed to join the circus.

Within our department, there was a balance of power between the "clinical" and the "research" wing. It was obvious that Dr. Braun made a great effort to keep out of the way of the Chairman of the Department and his research group. On the other hand, the Chairman reciprocated by giving Dr. Braun plenty of leeway in the clinical domain of the hospital. It was known that Dr. Braun had old ties with the Dean and the administration of the medical school. Besides that, the Chairman of the Department was not at all interested in the clinical practice of pathology. It was natural that the Chairman and the members of his research retinue cared for only one thing: obtaining large grants, to provide funding for research and for the benefit of the medical school.

While doing routine surgical diagnostic pathology, I also found time to do some research by using electron microscopes in the facilities of the academic group. In that way, I was working on both sides of an invisible divide between the academic and the clinical staff. I could not help to notice that there was a certain tension, a sort of competing attitude between Dr. Braun, together with the practicing physicians on one side, and the group of researchers who contributed to the medical school a great deal of funding on the other side.

Dr. Braun occasionally liked to refer to our researchers, only half in jest, as "the Mouseologists". This was a term that he invented, and he applied it to all scientists who did basic science research, regardless of whether they used mice or cats or no animals at all. The tone, with which Dr. Braun pronounced the word "Mouseologists," with the accent on the second "o," was also quite revealing, with a good dose of sarcasm and disdain. Although there was in the research wing of the medical school a whole floor housing a variety of animals for research, an area we called "the little zoo," Dr. Braun never had any use for it. His research was strictly clinical; he was a clinician and dealt only with patients.

In the course of time, I noticed that many members of our research group exuded a certain untoward attitude towards Dr. Braun, and, to some degree, also towards the entire clinical staff, those physicians who practiced with patients. That attitude could be best described as a "painful sufferance". Even within our own department, it appeared that some of the researchers looked upon us, practicing pathologists, with an elitist attitude that was not so subtle. It felt as if our practical work, providing pathologic diagnoses, were some sort of menial labor, whereas the basic science research was considered an endeavor requiring a superior, unique intellect, capable to reach the pinnacles of science. With such adversary vibes in the research labs, there were times when I, having received the courtesy of being allowed to work in the electron microscopy suite, felt as if I did not belong there... Perhaps it was only a badly constructed imagination, because, on a direct, personal level, everyone was very forthcoming and polite, and two of the researchers were old friends from the days of residency training.

Of course, Dr. Braun's feelings about "the Mouseologists" and "those clowns", as well as the researchers' elitist attitude towards the clinical staff - both struck me as offensive. Being the most junior in the department, I remained mute, and tried to ignore it, playing deaf and blind to all of it. So, I discovered that within a large department, one inevitably had to contend with the existence of ugly politics. I did not like any part of it, but since every coin has two sides, I had to use that worn-out coin very carefully, without looking too closely at either side of it.

Despite his persistent clinical research and numerous publications, Dr. Braun did not carry any grant from NIH or any similar agency. It was, however, widely known throughout our department that he received one of those special grants of 100,000 dollars that President Nixon awarded to 'deserving and important scientists' as a part of his "War on Cancer". With Nixon long gone, that "war," unfortunately, still goes on…

Each year, Dr. Braun used to take the whole month of August for his vacation, and during his absence, I had to perform a special part of his research. To be able to do that, he taught me an immunologic research procedure that was completely new to me. It was the "skin window technique," which Dr. Braun has been applying to all breast cancer patients of Dr. Larimer. Dr. Braun described the procedure as one where he could observe and study a patient's native cell reaction to her own cancer cells, whereby he could predict the prognosis of the patient's cancer.*

So it was that each year during the month of August, Dr. Larimer's patients would come to Dr. Braun's lab, and I would do the "skin window" test. The stained test material was saved till Dr. Braun came back from his vacation. He was the only one who knew how to interpret the patient's cell reaction, he kept his own records and shared the results with Dr. Larimer. In all those years, I was never shown how to "read" that cell reaction and make a prognosis of patient's cancer…

---

*"Skin window technique" was developed by John Rebuck in 1955. In Dr. Braun's application of this technique, the patient's own cancer cells were right after surgery preserved by making a cell smear on a plastic coverslip and saving it in a freezer. About one week later, the coverslip with cancer cells would be applied to the patient's skin on the inner side of the forearm, in an area where the top layer of skin was sharply abraded with a scalpel, to allow oozing of plasma fluid with white blood cells. That represented the "skin window". The coverslip with cancer cells was secured on the "window" with a Band-Aid, and it would remain there for 24 hours. The patient would come back the next day, and the coverslip would be removed and stained to study under the microscope the reaction between the patient's native white cells and her cancer cells.

In the mid-seventies, the hospitals were pressured to establish a "Quality Assessment Board," also known as the "Tumor Board," that is, a committee that reviewed and approved all research and therapeutic procedures for cancer conducted on hospital premises. Soon after the Tumor Board reviewed the "skin window" procedure, Dr. Braun stopped doing it. Some of our oncologists also had to stop using chemotherapy "cocktails" of their own invention, at least while practicing within the confines of the hospital. Only a few years ago, a public trial of a Michigan oncologist showed that this type of chemotherapy experimentation still occasionally takes place.

Within several years in an academic position, I published over a dozen clinical research papers directed toward making accurate pathologic diagnoses of various tumors and other conditions. Based on my research activity and the number of years as an Assistant Professor, I began to expect the customary promotion to the higher rank of Associate Professor. As this was not forthcoming, I brought up this issue with a friend in the research section of our department, and he promised to raise the question with the Chairman of the Department. A few days later, my friend let me know in great confidence that the Chairman had initiated my promotion already several months earlier but was waiting for it to be cleared by my immediate boss, Dr. Braun, who was still sitting on it. Hearing that, I became painfully aware that the research project Dr. Braun asked me to do soon after I joined the department has been still only "in progress".

I had to finalize the electron microscopic study of lymph gland reactions, which Dr. Braun's theory claimed could determine the prognosis of cancer. I had been working on that project, on and off, for years, but with great frustration. The work was difficult and unrewarding: at low magnifications, the electron microscopy showed the same cell patterns that could be seen with a light microscope, and thus provided no new information. At higher magnification, the electron microscopy showed a lot of fine detail within individual cells, but specific cell reaction patterns, as defined by Dr. Braun's theory, were no longer discernible. It was like seeing the detail of a single leaf but losing the sight of the whole tree. With such an impediment, there was no way that the electron microscopy could confirm the validity of Dr. Braun's theory. I decided to make a thorough description of each cell type found in the lymph nodes, without regard to cell pattern. I put together all my notes with data and all the best electron microscopic images that demonstrated the fine details of each cell type, and then took time to compose and write the paper, leaving out any indication about the prognosis of cancer, other than references to the previous papers of Dr. Braun.

One morning, I walked into Dr. Braun's office and, with great trepidation, handed him a typed copy of the paper with the electron images. Then I nervously attended to my daily work, all the while waiting for his response. By the early afternoon, I heard his heavy steps echoing through the hallway. He was on his way home. The next morning, as soon as I walked into his office and said, "Good morning", he looked up and brusquely said, "OK, let's publish it!"

I could see that he wasn't pleased. The paper was accepted for publication in a reputable journal, where Dr. Braun previously published many of his papers about lymph gland reaction to cancer. The publication went under my name, with Dr. Braun as co-author, and I added one more co-author, the assistant pathologist who helped me by doing the bulk of diagnostic work during the weeks I was preparing the manuscript.

Soon after the paper was published, I received a surprisingly large number of requests for a reprint, a sign that the publication was accepted with a lot of interest. (Mailing out reprints was the method of paper propagation in the seventies.) Then Dr. Braun began to show signs of satisfaction, mostly because there was so much interest in his theory, and perhaps a little bit also because it was the first time that he co-authored a paper that applied electron microscopy.

However, the interest in that paper was short-lived. Within a year after it was published, several reports came out from researchers who conducted retrospective light microscopic studies of lymph glands draining breast cancer. Their findings led to the conclusion that the cell reactions in those lymph glands were variable and inconsistent and, thus, could not be correlated with any specific prognosis. Over the next few years, Dr. Braun's theory remained a solitary hypothesis, and without further confirmation, it fell into oblivion.

The only positive thing that came out of publishing that paper was that my promotion to Associate Professor finally came through. With that, and with a total of ten years of experience in diagnostic pathology practice, my resume was well-rounded, and I was ready to seek the position of Director of Pathology in a good community hospital.

During my last one and a half years at the medical school, I was assigned an additional duty. When the Director of the Clinical Laboratory at the hospital suddenly retired, I was asked by the Chairman of the Department to step into his position. Along with my regular work, I then had to supervise the entire clinical laboratory. With experience in directing clinical labs, this new duty did not give me any trouble, especially because the lab was well organized and had an experienced technical staff. As a fun part of that job, I supervised the very first introduction of a relatively new technology, the radioimmunoassay (RIA) in our lab. It was first applied to measure the thyroid hormone levels and then the hormone levels of other glands with internal secretion.

Acting as Director of a large hospital laboratory gave me a good overview of changes regarding the personnel running medical laboratories. Through political manipulation, the senior laboratory technologists had lobbied for and managed to promulgate a regulation that allowed them to obtain the title of 'Director of Laboratory' issued by the local Department of Health. The title was based on lab experience of ten or more years, commonly called "the grandfather clause". So long as the laboratory did only chemical, hematologic and bacteriologic testing, a senior technologist could be promoted to Director of Laboratory. If the lab received any tissue biopsies or cytology samples, it had to have a pathologist certified in Anatomic Pathology.

Thus, the pathologists and their expertise would soon become superfluous in running an average medical laboratory. Using medical technologists as directors, the laboratory services became less costly and left more profit to the owners. In the next several years, through mergers and acquisitions, the medical laboratory services in the US were reduced to a handful of giant laboratories, forming a network of branches that served practically the entire country. Of course, there are still about 200,000 small independent local medical laboratories, but their capacity is unable to cover the extreme demands during a national emergency or a pandemic. And yet, despite great progress in technology, with the bulk of routine testing being run on large, automated and computerized equipment, with a minimal amount of chemicals and very little labor, the cost of lab tests has been steadily rising. That may be credited to the clever management of profit.

The Lab Manager at the medical school hospital, Mr. Porter was one of those senior technologists who was recently "grandfathered" to the rank of Director of Laboratory. He felt that having a pathologist as Director of the Laboratory was an imposition. He did not know that I was soon to leave the hospital and take on a new position. About a month prior to my leaving, I submitted my resignation to the Chairman of the Department and felt that it was time to notify the Lab Manager and the supervisors of various lab sections. Just then, Mr. Porter had called a special meeting of all members of laboratory staff, and I thought, it would be a perfect occasion to make the announcement of my imminent departure.

When I quietly entered the meeting room, there was a sudden silence, as if my appearance was of some special importance. I greeted everyone and asked the Lab Manager for permission to make a short announcement. Mr. Porter kindly allowed me to speak, and I simply told all present technologists and supervisors that I would soon be leaving the medical school and taking on a new position out of town and thanked them for their help and excellent services during my tenure as Director. I received congratulations and good wishes, and soon, I excused myself and left the meeting. Later that day, one of the lab supervisors approached me and let me know that Mr. Porter had called that meeting with the sole purpose of soliciting the lab personnel to sign a petition to the Chairman of the Department, asking him to remove me from the position of director and instead, appoint Mr. Porter.

During the entire first year in my new position as Director of Pathology and Laboratory in a community hospital away from NYC, I continued my contact with the medical school and managed to visit and even give two lectures to medical students. That same year, the medical school moved to a new campus with a new modern hospital. The sad news was that the old academic hospital, well-known and respected in NYC for many decades, was closed, and it was later refurbished to serve for other purposes.

Chapter 10

The Joys of a Director of Pathology and Laboratory

At the end of June of 1977, I rented a small apartment in a little city in the North-East of US. The apartment was within walking distance from the hospital where I accepted the position of Director of Pathology and Laboratory. The area was in a little valley, carved out by a river, with a string of small towns, all connected to one another and surrounded by green hills and adjacent rural areas. The region housed several important industrial facilities, which I soon found were liable to cause major pollution of the local water supply.

Several colleges and universities in the region offered occasional cultural events, and a not-too-distant small mountain provided reasonably good skiing facilities, a worthy asset in an area where winters lasted at least seven months, and ten-foot-high snow piles could firmly persist around the edges of a driveway, to melt only by the first week of May.

My family remained for the summer in our New York suburban home, which Miriam had put up for sale. After a full day's work, living away from the family, I went out every night for dinner. Sampling the various restaurants in the area was fun, and I found that they all presented healthy home cuisine with lots of local farm products. All the restaurants had one rather unusual offering in common: an enormous mound of large shrimp was a regular part of the salad bar, which came for free with the dinner. I liked the shrimp, and often, by the time I got my main course, I could hardly eat any more. I certainly never managed to have a dessert. At the end of summer, by the time my family arrived in town, we bought a house, but we still often went out for dinner. Our whole family enjoyed the free salad bar with shrimp.

Within about nine months, there was a sudden change in all local restaurants. They still had the free salad bar included with dinner, but the best item in the salad had disappeared. The mound of shrimp was no longer present. Being new in the area, I was regularly reading the local newspapers, and it was there that I saw an interesting article, fully explaining the disappearance of shrimp from the salads. The article came under a curious title: *"A two-year-old puzzle is finally solved!"* and here follows a summary of it.

For the past two years, it was noticed that whole truckloads of seafood have been mysteriously disappearing from the largest fish market on the East Coast, the Fulton Fish Market in NYC. The authorities had finally tracked down the disappearing seafood to a cold storage facility in our region. The owner of the facility claimed that he frequently received seafood shipments for cold storage without an initial downpayment. The customers usually paid when they came to pick up the stored items. The depositors, in some cases, failed to pick up their merchandise, no storage payments were ever made, and after three months passed without any compensation, the owner was compelled to sell the stored items at a nominal cost just to cover his expenses. The owner of the cold storage gave the police all basic information about the depositors: the names and addresses of the companies that owned and delivered the merchandise. He did not personally know all his clients. Unfortunately, the authorities could never find any of the recorded clients' companies at the listed addresses. The owner of the cold storage facility was warned that in the future, he would be held fully responsible for verifying the authenticity of all his depositors and clients…

This was happening during that strange period between 1977 and 1981, a time when deep social and economic changes were taking shape. At work, what I used to know as the Personnel Department, had been renamed into the "Department of Human Resources" (HR), and I had to get adjusted to thinking of myself as a sort of commodity. Like everyone else, I learned to adjust and accept it. After all, the janitors have been transformed into "superintendents", and the garbage collectors into "sanitation workers". Even the good old meaning of a nice, innocent and happy word (gay!) had acquired a new, completely different meaning... But let's not worry about words, because a much more important economic change took place: the explosive inflation. Some said that it was promulgated by the government's fiscal actions to help the economy. The inflation and the interest rates were not only in the double digits, but for a while as high as fourteen percent, and at one brief point in 1980, they reached as high as 18! Yes, that was eighteen percent!

The town we came to live in had at that time an unusually talented mayor. The local industries were polluting the drinking water to a point where one or another local water well had to be put out of circulation, to be cleaned. It would take six months to a year to clean out a polluted well. On some occasions, the local residents were advised to avoid drinking water from their faucets. Plenty of bottled water was available in the stores. It is not necessary to name the powerful major companies involved in pollution, and anyway, more than one industry took part, as if it were a competition. When the mayor was asked why the companies were not fined and ordered to stop the pollution, he gave an answer that was truly candid: "The town could not afford to risk damaging its tax base." And who could object to such an honest answer?

Only a couple of years later, there was a new mayor, and it happened again: the water well in one town was suddenly found so polluted that the citizens were advised to avoid taking hot showers. The vapors were too toxic! That new mayor went to attend a conference of mayors in Washington DC but failed to notice that it was a conference of Democrat mayors. Ours was a Republican. Nevertheless, our local paper reported that the mayor was cordially received by the Democrats and returned home "full of cheer..."

Periodically, we could read in the local news that an industrial plant "accidentally released" some toxic material directly into the local river. Since the region was known for its nearly 300 cloudy days in a year and was endowed with abundant rainfall (they compared it with Belgium), it was felt that the river would eventually flush all the toxins into the ocean, and our local pollution problem would go away.

And soon thereafter, a tidbit in the local newspaper informed us that it was the 50th anniversary of the day when the KKK burned a cross on a little hill where our house was located. At least by then, the KKK was long gone from the area, chased away by a local industrialist who employed a lot of Catholic people from Eastern Europe and did not appreciate the attitude of the KKK towards his workers. Looking a little deeper into the local history, one could also find examples of how the new settlers dealt with the Native Americans, who had either "moved away" or entirely disappeared. When one comes to live in a new region, it is important to learn its history, whether glorious or not.

We wanted our four children to attend the public schools. For the two in grade school, we were not too disturbed by the occasional loss of a warm winter jacket; there were some needy people in the area. But our two children in junior high school came home telling us of a serious disorder in classes. The teachers were spending more time to keep order than to do some teaching. The English teacher never assigned the students a list of books to read, and when Miriam inquired about it, the teacher's reaction was:

"Well, the kids really don't like reading. We are happy if they read the comics!" Then followed some dangerous incidents: fires were set by students in the school locker rooms or in the bathrooms. When the frequency of those fires became a weekly event, especially in winter, and the students were rushed out into the freezing air on the street without proper clothing, we decided to send our two older children to a private school. They both graduated from the local Catholic High School.

After a few years, we found that one of the local towns had a 'somewhat better' public school, and we sold our house and moved to a home in that town. That way, our two younger children graduated from a public school. But before they graduated, they came home with stories about certain classmates dealing drugs, and teachers who quietly looked the other way, not daring to say anything, simply out of fear. And then, one day, there was the story about a student who brought to school a firebomb, right into the class. Luckily, the teacher caught him in time and quickly grabbed the bomb and threw it out the window. The next moment they all heard the explosion. And so, we too received an education about the 'good' rural schools.

*   *   *

And my new job? The new position? Let's just say that the first few months of being a Director of Pathology and Laboratory in a local community hospital were quite challenging, and no less exciting. The hospital administrator, Mr. Loughlin and the Medical Director, Dr. Blusher let me know on the very first day that my predecessor, Dr. Smith had been asked to leave because he was, as they put it, "not paying attention to the requirements of his job". They also advised me that the remaining Assistant Pathologist, was also considered "unfit for his position" and that I should dismiss him as soon as I am able to find a satisfactory replacement. That request I wanted to postpone, at least, till I had a chance to evaluate him by myself.

Within the first week on the job, I learned from several members of the laboratory staff that my predecessor, Dr. Smith, had served as director of the department for 18 full years, and I overheard one of the technologists say: "… and it was a shame that he had to leave." Was it deliberately said within my earshot? Maybe not, but it sure gave me a message. Besides, I heard from others in the hospital some lovely expressions, like: "Dr. Smith was a good local man," and "a charming person," and "truly beloved by everyone in the hospital." He owned a dairy farm with over one hundred heads of cows, and he was currently taking care of his farm. I was new in the area, new to the job, and apparently, I had a steep hill to climb to measure up to my predecessor. At times, I felt somewhat anxious: how will I fit in? I owned no cows, nor was I a "charming local."

Aside from routinely performing day-to-day diagnostic service in surgical pathology, one of my primary tasks was to immediately assess the fiscal performance of the clinical laboratory, as well as the staff and equipment. The Assistant Pathologist, Dr. Som Saetan was a few years older than I, very pleasant and friendly, and he tried to make himself as helpful as he could. He introduced me to the laboratory staff and shared with me the routine daily diagnostic work. Within the first week of my arrival, Dr. Blusher, the Medical Director, called me one morning and told me to come right after lunch, at 1 pm, into his office. He explained that I was to meet "a highly respected surgeon", Dr. Adam Konig, an ENT specialist. Dr. Blusher further informed me, that Dr. Konig, unfortunately, during the past year, completely stopped admitting his patients to our hospital. The purpose of the meeting was to introduce me to Dr. Konig, and to persuade him that with a new pathologist on board, he should resume admitting his patients into our hospital. Hearing that, I felt like a new dish in an old restaurant.

I walked into Dr. Blusher's office a few minutes ahead of time, anxious to hear some more about this Dr. Konig. No chance! Dr. Konig appeared at the door within less than a minute. A stocky man with dark hair and lively brown eyes, he looked at me and extended his hand with a firm grip:

"Adam Konig, glad to meet you!"

Dr. Blusher introduced me, and while I offered Dr. Konig my hand, he kept measuring me up and down and said:

"So, you are the new pathologist!" and he sat on a chair offered by Dr. Blusher. I sat down next to Dr. Blusher, and Dr. Konig again turned to me with a mischievous look and said:

"You know, your predecessor used to provide me with 'Mickey Mouse' diagnoses!"

I looked at him, perplexed, while Dr. Blusher just smiled. Dr. Konig went on:

"Well, let's say that those diagnoses did not make much sense, you know, just like something Mickey Mouse would tell you!"

"Aaah!" I gasped, beginning to understand. After ten years of practicing pathology in NYC, I came far into the hinterland and just learned an entirely new term, apparently invented by an ENT surgeon for a doubtful or simply wrong diagnosis. I gathered myself together and said:

"I promise you will not get any 'Mickey Mouse' diagnosis from me! Mickey will be kept out of my department!" Dr. Blusher immediately added:

"You see! We eliminated the problem!"

Dr. Konig stood up, turned to Dr. Blusher, and said:

"Well, I will start bringing in my patients!" and then, turning to me with a big smile, he declared, half menacing:

"I am going to test you!"

Our meeting was over. In a brisk, busy manner, Dr. Konig said a quick "goodbye" and walked out the door. Through the following years, he and I got to know each other quite well. We frequently met and enjoyed each other's company outside the hospital and, together with our wives, developed a wonderful, lasting friendship.

In the laboratory, the equipment was the easiest part to assess, and within two weeks, I surveyed the entire inventory and the lab's budget. To my great consternation, I found that the lab functioned as a big "cost center" instead of being, as normally expected, a revenue center. The lab had on lease an automated chemistry analyzer that was supposed to do a standard series of 20 most common tests at a nominal cost of 4 dollars per patient for the chemical reagents. However, this analyzer was totally unstable and gave out test results that were too unreliable to be reported. For all practical purposes, the analyzer was unusable, but its three-year lease agreement, signed only six months earlier, could not be cancelled. As a remedy, the staff was routinely using a machine that could do only one single test at a time, and the cost for each individual chemistry test kit was about 3.50 dollars. This latter machine had been designed by DuPont Company specifically for emergency situations when only one or two single test results were quickly needed. The machine was not developed for routine daily use, which requires a battery of 20 tests per patient. One did not need to be a math whizz to see that the routine chemistry series of tests run on the emergency analyzer cost the hospital 70 dollars per patient (20 x 3.50) instead of only 4 dollars. The excessive use of the emergency analyzer cost the hospital a total of 10-12,000 dollars per month, just for the patented individual test kits, not counting the cost of increased labor, as the technologists had to constantly "feed" the machine with hundreds of single test kits, one after the other. The hospital held the dubious record of being the largest single user of DuPont chemical kits in the Northeast! The current Lab Manager, apparently, did not see anything wrong with this type of operation.

When I asked, who chose the automated chemistry equipment for the lab, the Lab Manager blamed Dr. Smith. From documentation, it was obvious that it was the Lab Manager, who actively participated in assessing and choosing the lab equipment, though Dr. Smith did sign off on the final approval. There would soon be growing evidence that the Lab Manager also lacked the expected technical skills and knowledge required in his position. Whenever he had to step in for an absent lab section supervisor, he was unable to direct the technologists in proper running and maintenance of the equipment, and I would be called to straighten the problem.

From his resume, I found that the Lab Manager received "on-the-job training" while serving in the Army, and upon discharge, he somehow obtained the certificate of a lab technologist. However, he did have considerable other managerial talents: he was the chief regional salesman for Amway, and in that capacity, the hospital allowed him to hold monthly sales of Amway merchandise to hospital employees. Then I made a more disturbing discovery: the Lab Manager was hired by and was a protege of the Chief of HR, to whom he gave each day a ride to work and back home. This was a convenient arrangement because the Chief of HR had suffered an accident that left him with very poor vision, to the extent that he could not hold a driver's license.

After about six weeks on the job, I was able to present to the hospital administration a thorough review of the departmental budget, with equipment and personnel assessment. The excessive lab costs (instead of income!) were a red flag, and this was a problem. I presented the remedies: different lab equipment that would be immediately cost-effective and a new, better-qualified Manager. My recommendations about new chemistry equipment were immediately taken to be studied by the "central purchasing administration", which acted for a group of over 30 associated hospitals. The present Lab Manager would have to be confronted with a detailed list of his deficiencies and asked to resign or be dismissed. Considering his liaison with the Chief of HR, I had to go easy and carefully document all the facts.

There came a morning when I confronted the Lab Manager and gave him a printed list of his deficiencies. He quickly read the list and then, very eloquently, met me with a categorical denial of all his failings, including a sharp display of hostility. I sent a copy of his deficiencies to Mr. Loughlin, the hospital administrator responsible for the laboratory. A day after he was confronted with his deficiencies, the Lab Manager came to work wearing a very large Christ on a Cross, conspicuously hanging over the middle of his chest. Was I perhaps supposed to be intimidated by this sudden display of religiosity? The Cross became a permanent part of his attire. The Chief of Human Resources soon called me for a meeting, wanting to know what the problem was with the Lab Manager. I met him briefly, and referred him to the Hospital Administrator, Mr. Loughlin, who had the written documentation and would make the final decision.

The Lab Manager resigned, and during the next twelve and a half years, I had to contend with a Chief of HR, who lost his free driver and was not at all a friend. I let a few months go before promoting an experienced lab technologist to the position of Lab Manager. The new manager lacked a few credentials but made it up by taking correspondence courses in lab technology and management. It also helped that she was a "local". She was diligent and prudent and stayed in that position for the remaining 12 years I served as Director.

However, over the time, I learned that a manager's ultimate loyalty belongs to hospital administration, and not to the director of laboratory. Nevertheless, she always treated me with care, courtesy and respect.

The chemistry section of the laboratory required prompt action to eliminate losses from its poorly chosen analyzer. To that end, I proposed to obtain three small, relatively inexpensive pieces of equipment that would perform the required 20 tests per patient in the most economical way. That equipment could later always serve as a back-up to a large, automated machine. I sent a copy of the order for the proposed equipment to a sales representative who I knew from NYC, and his proposal arrived within a few days. After a couple of weeks, I also received a copy of the invoice from the "central purchasing administration" and discovered that their price was higher than the quote from NYC. The group purchasing agency acting for over 30 hospitals and located in the Midwest surely handled much larger orders than a single agent in NYC, and yet, they were going to pay a higher price for the same equipment! I decided it was better not to try to outdo the mighty "central purchasing", and I told the sales rep in NYC that the hospital got a "better deal".

As forewarned, I quickly found that the Assistant Pathologist, Dr. Saetan, lacked a solid training in pathology. He was not in the habit of reading professional journals, nor had he attended in the past several years any of the annual pathology meetings and courses to keep up with new developments. Now follows one not-so-amusing incident that happened within two months of my arrival.

One morning, Dr Saetan received a thick needle core biopsy from a breast tumor for a rapid frozen section diagnosis. He walked into my office, handed me a microscopic slide, and said:

"I got a frozen section from a breast tumor; please, look at it! It's a very strange tumor... I have never seen this before!"

"Well, let's see!" and I put the slide under my microscope and looked at it for a few seconds. In disbelief, I moved my head back and then took a quick second look and, without a word, grabbed the phone. While Dr. Saetan was still standing next to me, I dialed the operating room and asked to speak to Dr. Kraft, a senior surgeon who sent the biopsy. He expected the call and responded immediately, but since he was on a speakerphone that everyone in the operating room could hear, I asked him to take off his gloves, get out of the room, and call me back on the private line in the doctors' lounge. When he called, I asked:

"Is your patient very skinny?"

"Yes, she is, very! How did you know?"

"You've got a solid core biopsy of the myocardium!" and Dr. Kraft gasped:

"Ooh, my... The needle went that deep. Aah..., thank you!" and he hung up to quickly return to the patient. Further surgery on the breast tumor was postponed for another day. The patient was under anesthesia, and there was no ill-effect. I, however, was left quite perturbed. Finding that Dr. Saetan did not recognize under the microscope a piece of the normal heart muscle and that he mistook it for a "strange tumor" gave me an instant explanation why the hospital administration wanted him dismissed and replaced by a better-qualified pathologist.

A few days later, I received an urgent call from Dr. Maguire, the Chairman of Obstetrics and Gynecology. Upset and furious, he was screaming at me through the phone receiver, irate about an apparently erroneous pathologic diagnosis made on a placenta:

"The baby was born dead!" he yelled so loud that I had to hold the receiver a foot from my ear. He continued, "And it bled out from the broken vessels in the membrane! And your diagnosis says that the placenta was normal! How can that be?"

"My diagnosis?"

"Well, it was Dr. Saetan's, but it's your department!"

"I will check it out and send you my report, right away!"

"Check it out! And I need a corrected report! Thank you!" and he hung up. I immediately went to personally examine that placenta. I asked Tina, the technician who usually helped with the gross examination and cutting of pathology specimens, to find the container and show me the placenta.

When she opened the container, there was a deformed placenta with large abnormal blood vessels running across its thin membrane, with a tear of the vessels at the margin where the membrane was ruptured during baby's delivery. I asked:

"Tina, does Dr. Saetan examine the placentas and measure and weigh them by himself, or do you, maybe, do it for him?"

She hesitated for a moment, and then answered:

"No, no, he does it!"

Tina blushed. She had known and worked with Dr. Saetan for a good number of years. He was a kind and likable person, and naturally, she tried to cover up for him. She appeared embarrassed. I went to my office, dictated a new report, had it immediately typed, signed it, and had it sent out to the patient's chart, with a copy to Dr. Maguire's office.

Then I did some quick thinking: *Did Dr. Saetan look at that placenta too quickly and carelessly fail to see the abnormality in the membrane, or did he never even see it, but let Tina open the container and record the measurements and weight?* The answer to the question did not matter at all! One thing was sure: our department issued a "Mickey Mouse" diagnosis. This time, I would promptly have to follow exactly what the administrators suggested on my first day of work. It was "the last straw", and Dr. Saetan would have to go and find employment somewhere else.

Within half an hour, I called him into my office, and he came with his head hanging. I could see that he sensed what was coming. Tina must have told him of my inquiry. We had a frank discussion, and it was hard… Never before have I been the boss and director of the department, and never have I been in a position where I had to dismiss another attending pathologist. Dr. Saetan agreed to resign and said he would immediately start looking for a job. Times had changed: suddenly, there seemed to be a slight oversupply of pathologists, except in some more remote parts of the country. I let him have three months' time to find a position.

First thing the next morning, I received a call from Sr. Amalia, an Assistant Administrator, and she asked me to come for a brief meeting in her office. As soon as I walked in, she said:

"Dr. Yellinek, I received a very serious complaint from Dr. Maguire! Your department made a grievous error in diagnosis!"

I explained that I already issued a corrected diagnosis, and it should immediately clarify the cause of the infant's death. This was one of those rare events where abnormally developed blood vessels grew across the placental membrane and were ruptured during delivery; the baby bled out before the delivery was completed. It was clearly not the fault of Dr. Maguire. Wanting to end this unpleasant meeting, I said:

"I already spoke to Dr. Saetan, and he has resigned. He served here for nine years, and considering his family with four children, I gave him three months to find a job."

"Dr. Yellinek," and Sr. Amalia spoke with a very friendly, soft, and soothing tone, like talking to a child, slowly annunciating and pausing between every few words, "you are now… a Director of a Department. You now have to… think with your head… and not with your heart!" Then she looked me in the eyes, and suddenly continued with a cold, hard, angry tone, as if it were coming from another person, sounding like an army sergeant:

"Dr. Saetan must clear out of his office and leave the hospital by the end of THIS day!"

"I understand! I will let him know!"

Our brief meeting ended quickly, and I went to my office to sit in my chair and calm down. After a few minutes, I went to Dr. Saetan's office and said:

"Som, I am sorry! The administration wants you to leave today, at the end of the day. I cannot do anything! You know, there were issues before I came…"

"I know…"

"I hope they will let you have the severance pay, I mean, the three months of salary."

That same afternoon, right after lunch, a hospital security guard came to the pathology department to watch and assist Dr. Saetan with gathering and packing up his possessions.

This was the first important lesson I received as a Director of Pathology, and it was delivered so very effectively by a young nun, a manager in training… It took Dr. Saetan about two and a half months to find a job in a Veterans' Administration Hospital, somewhere in the South. Our hospital did pay his salary for three months, and that made me feel a little better.

Meanwhile, I had met several pathologists from the hospital in a neighboring town and managed to hire one of them away to become my assistant.

As the dust from my first encounters as Director started to settle, I began to see the larger picture within and around the hospital. While the administrators were dealing with day-to-day issues, Dr. Blusher, the Medical Director was aiding the hospital to achieve better efficiency in collecting reimbursement for its services. At the end of the seventies and through the eighties, the hospitals were being increasingly pressured by the insurance industry to shorten the length of stay (LOS) of the in-patients and to accomplish various other efficiencies, including the performance of minor surgery and some other procedures in the clinic, without overnight patient admission to the hospital.

Over the next few years, Dr. Blusher recruited two consulting firms which conducted interminable interviews with everyone and anyone in the hospital. Two months later, after having paid a substantial fee, the hospital received a thick book with survey results, findings, and a list of recommendations. Some of the recommendations were logical and good, but many were impossible to apply. One of the consulting firms was invited to teach each hospital department how to do the "correct coding" of diagnoses. The coding had to be "maximized", and to achieve that goal, one had to apply "creative methods". All these measures were taken with the aim of improving the desperately needed reimbursements.

The consulting firms were handsomely profiting from the fact that many hospital administrators and their finance chiefs were endowed with a good dose of incompetence. The news all over the press at that time was that Washington, DC, was swarming with consultants of all kinds. It was a national trend, and it was augmented by the ignorance of individuals who were in charge of various companies and enterprises. CEOs and managers, who may have had a knack for politicking sufficient to obtain their position and salary, were simply not capable of performing their jobs. Hiring a consultant, the managers and CEOs would try to defer their problems and shift the responsibility for any failure onto the consultants.

Dr. Blusher took time to attend a well-known Management Course given by Harvard University, and he brought with him a copy of an inch thick manual for hospital perusal. As a director of a department, I received a copy and really benefitted from studying the entire course. It taught me all the professional terms and names for various management acts and methods, many of which I had been applying as a matter of common sense. It also taught me about the long history of management, starting with the example of how the Egyptian pyramids were built by clever management of slaves. Among other things, I still remember learning for the first time the term and the meaning of "self-actualization". It was such a complicated, long word, a whole mouthful. I read the entire chapter about it and understood well the concept of it, though I would never have to worry about it.

Self-actualization, if it were ever achieved, would be attained mostly by quite accomplished people, and certainly somewhat later in life, closer to the time of retirement. Only a few exceptional people or geniuses might attain it much earlier. I was at that time nowhere near it and did not want to even begin to think about it. Most people are happily unaware of it, and its absence doesn't do them any harm.

Dr. Blusher also brought to the hospital a consultant who was "an expert in word use", one who even wrote a book about "the real meaning" of words. His presentation and lecture were quite interesting: he tried to go as far as teaching how one may "honestly" justify giving the answer "yes", when it should be understood that it meant "no", and vice versa. He might as well have described his book as being about the false meaning of words. This muddling of the meaning of words made me remember how our press famously reported that Khrushchev had agreed to some US proposal by clearly saying "Da, da" (= yes, yes), and then it was a surprise, a real scandal, when he firmly denied that he ever agreed to that proposal. Our translators failed to catch the meaning of a double "yes" in Russian language. Such gymnastics with words may be useful in politics and diplomacy, but as a pathologist, I had no use for obfuscation. I needed to tell only simple, straight facts to make clear diagnostic statements. As for the management of personnel, I knew enough to tactfully say "maybe" or "let's think about it" and avoid a false and deceitful "yes" or "no". Every parent knows to apply that method managing children. To bluntly say "no" when one knew that the answer was "yes" was an outright falsehood, a plain deception commonly practiced by certain types of people, including diplomats and politicians. I had little use for any of that lecture, and I had absolutely no regard for this type of "real meaning" of words. That lecture was a typical ploy for professional managers, a lecture on how to deceive and manipulate people.

Then, one year Dr. Blusher attended a meeting in Chicago, where a group of 'experts' in healthcare presented the "proper criteria for doing surgery". Those criteria were published in a book with a bright red cover, and after returning from Chicago, Dr. Blusher gave me a copy to look it over. He suggested that I should study those criteria for surgery, and since, as a pathologist I get to see all the products of surgery, I should be able to persuade our staff surgeons to adopt and implement the principles of those criteria in their practice. Dr. Blusher maintained that adhering to those criteria would improve the quality of hospital services and would thereby bring a better reimbursement rate to the hospital. After carefully reading that book, I quickly realized that the criteria for doing surgery were written so narrowly that more than half the procedures done at any hospital would be deemed unnecessary and disallowed and not paid for. The people who compiled the book, obviously had their minds bent on cutting the expenses of the medical insurance industry, with the least concern for the patients' health or the quality of care. It appeared that Dr. Blusher's own philosophy agreed with the agenda of the people who wrote the book. On this subject, I dragged my feet and avoided meeting Dr. Blusher for as long as I could. Meanwhile, I showed the book to my friend Dr. Laporta, the chief of thoracic surgery, and then we both carefully surveyed the last twenty of his operations. When we applied the book's criteria, it turned out that in fully one-half of the cases, the operation would be disallowed, even though all the procedures were necessary and clearly beneficial to the patients.

Finally, the day came when Dr. Blusher called me to have a formal meeting about the subject of the red book. At the meeting, I simply told him that based on what Dr. Laporta and I found, we should not recommend to our surgeons to apply the criteria from that book. Dr. Blusher became visibly upset and retorted with an irritated tone:

"Are you refusing to follow my recommendation?"

"No, no! I only mean that someone else would be better suited to persuade the surgeons to implement the…" He cut me off:

"These criteria are good! I know it! And it is the task of the pathologist to put it through! This is important for the hospital!"

"I do respect your opinion, but I am sorry! As a pathologist, I don't have the expertise to tell the surgeons when they may or may not do an operation. I am not in a position to do it!"

"Well..." and he raised his voice, "...as Medical Director of the hospital, I am giving you an order to do it! You better think it over!"

"Yes, Dr. Blusher, I'll think about—" but he again cut me off:

"OK then! You'll let me know how it's going."

"Is there a deadline for this?"

"I leave it up to you!"

On this calmer note, our meeting was over. But later that day, I thought about it and concluded that Dr. Blusher was my boss, and he had the right to give me orders, but this last order was wrong. His manner was threatening, and this order went beyond the limit of reasonable...

As Dr. Blusher suggested, I thought a little more about it. To go up against a powerful Medical Director who participated in hiring me, would not be a good thing. But by then, I had been Director of Pathology for three years, and I felt that I was well accepted by the medical staff and by other hospital executives, except for the chief of HR. I decided that it was time to go discuss the whole issue with the head administrator of the hospital. She was a wise and experienced senior nun who I formally met and spoke to only a few times. Within one day, I got an appointment, and at the given time, I appeared in her office. She offered me a seat, and I briefly presented the essence of my conflict with Dr. Blusher. My position was that I could not recommend the excessively stringent criteria to our surgeons. By that time, I also heard that Dr. Blusher had given a copy of the red book to his friend, the Director of Pathology in a hospital in the neighboring town, and that the surgeons in that hospital made an uproar when that pathologist tried to suggest that they use those criteria for surgery. They wouldn't have any part of it! I told all of this to the head administrator, and she listened very attentively. I decided the night before the meeting that to put an end to the ugly clash with Dr. Blusher, I would have to go on a limb, and I said:

"I do not mean any disrespect for Dr. Blusher, but if my reluctance to get involved in this issue were to remain a problem, I would have to offer my resignation…"

The head administrator just smiled:

"I don't think it will have to come to that! I need to speak to Dr. Blusher. I want to hear his side, and then, all three of us will meet and discuss it."

"Thank you for your time."

"You are welcome, and God bless!"

When that meeting ended, I was quite relieved, but I knew that the whole issue still had to be resolved.

So, I had the first serious crisis in my job as Director. Three long days later, I was called to come to a meeting at the head administrator's office. As I entered the room, I saw, to my dismay, that Dr. Blusher was already sitting there, and his face wore a stiff grin. I felt instantly tense and anxious, and it must have shown on me too. As soon as I took a chair, the head administrator, with a calm voice came straight to the point:

"Well, it's good that we all meet. We decided… that you, Dr. Yellinek, should continue to follow Dr. Blusher's lead in all matters, just as you've always been doing. Well, now… in the case of these criteria for surgery…, right now both of you should best set all this aside and let it cool down! And for now, let's give that red book a little rest and put it up on a shelf! But you two…, you should now shake hands on it, and continue to work nicely together, as you always did!"

"Yes, we will!" we both said almost in unison, and the two of us got up and shook hands. It was obvious that the administrator talked to Dr. Blusher well before I joined the meeting, and she must have indicated to him that at least "for now," it would be best to "sit on it" for a while…

My first big crisis was resolved by a wise nun/administrator, and the 'red book' was left to rest on a shelf. This issue was somehow forgotten, and it was never brought up again. As for Dr. Blusher, my communication with him was henceforth always careful, concise, and correct. Afterwards, I noticed that in my presence he never smiled, and usually carried only a broad grin. We had a truce, though with a palpable tension, and both of us learned to live with it for the next nine years. We did have occasional brief moments of a thaw, but never a complete relaxation. With Dr. Blusher, one had better always be on guard!

Chapter 11

Oncology

Oncology is defined as the study of tumors, and it is also the name of a hospital department that deals with the treatment of cancer. I was Director of Pathology in a general hospital that served as a regional cancer center, with a strong department of oncology and radiation therapy. There, I had the opportunity to see a great variety of tumors and to continue with clinical research on cancer. As soon as I settled in my position, I joined the ECOG (Eastern Cooperative Oncology Group), a large nationwide group of oncologists and pathologists that had the purpose of reviewing thousands of cases of various cancers from across the whole country to provide a reliable diagnostic standard. Since the oncologists developed precise protocols for the treatment of every subtype of cancer, it was of utmost importance to have an absolutely accurate pathologic diagnosis of each cancer variant (subtype), so that a proper protocol of therapy could be applied. My participation at ECOG was concentrated in two specific sections: cancer of the breast and cancer (sarcoma) of bone, joints and connective tissues. Those cancer types had, in the previous ten years, become the subject of my special interest and study.

ECOG functioned mostly by mail: the microscopic slides of cancer cases were regularly mailed back and forth between the member pathologists to be reviewed according to set diagnostic criteria. The reviewers' diagnostic reports were mailed to the ECOG management center at the University of Madison, in Madison, WI. The member pathologists were located all over the US, and a few were in several countries in Europe. Once a year, the pathologists would travel to

Madison, WI, to spend a week in meetings and lectures, coordinating and improving their skills in cancer diagnosis. In addition, twice a year, I would meet for a full day's work with a group of pathologists working on tumors of bone and connective tissue, either in Philadelphia, PA, or in Springfield, MA, where the group leaders resided.

At the 1979 ECOG meeting in Madison, WI, it was announced that a pathologist had submitted a proposal asking ECOG to adopt a new cell grading system for breast cancer, which he had developed over the past 20 years. With this proposal, ECOG received a set of microscopic slides of breast cancer, with each slide marked as a typical example of one of the three distinct cell grades. Following scientific principles, the evaluation of the slides would be done blindly by the senior members of the Pathology Department at the University of Madison. As with all blind evaluations, the names of the evaluators and of the submitting pathologist were not revealed, and all results were to be sorted out by independent statisticians.

While working closely with the ECOG center in Madison, WI, I was periodically kept abreast with all new developments, and a few months later, there was a follow-up about the newly proposed breast cancer cell grading. The blind evaluation study of the submitted microscopic slides ended with significant discrepancies between the findings of the reviewers in Madison. The team of evaluators decided to try a different approach: they invited the submitting pathologist to Madison and asked him to personally demonstrate on a set of microscopic slides with breast cancer, how to correctly classify each cell grade in his system. At the next ECOG meeting in Madison, in 1980, there was a result for the proposed breast cancer grading system, and below is the interesting summary of it:

EVALUATION OF GRADING SYSTEM FOR BREAST CANCER CELLS

A) METHOD

1. The submitting pathologist's own original slides are disguised by replacing his labels with Madison U. labels with a coded grade.

2. The pathologist will thus blindly grade his own slides for the second time.

3. If correctly graded, the procedure will prove that the grading system is reproducible.

B) STATISTICAL RESULT AND CONCLUSION

1. Repeat grading of the same slides differed significantly from the original.

2. The submitting pathologist did not reproduce his own grading correctly.

3. The grading system lacks reproducibility and is not acceptable.

After reading the report, I asked one of the ECOG principals in Madison if it was possible to know the name of the member who proposed the new grading of breast cancer cells. He did not know it but promised to look it up. The next day, before the meeting started, he brought me a piece of paper with the name of the pathologist: Morton Braun, MD, Professor of Pathology.

This was not a surprise. What I quietly suspected during years of working under Dr. Braun, was finally confirmed by the ECOG team. His newly invented breast cancer cell grading was inconsistent and unusable. His theory of specific lymph node reactions to cancer, his interpretation of skin window immune reaction, and all his prognostic prophecies were a product of his own rich imagination. He kept repeating his theories for years, he talked about them on and on, he managed to publish multiple papers on the same subject, and he forced us, the pathologists in his department, to add to all the official diagnostic reports a coded footnote with his invented cell grades and lymph gland reactions. He must have deeply believed in his theories, and since no one dared to contradict him, he was able to continue with that whole act.

Shortly after I returned home from that ECOG meeting, I wanted to check out something that I had been curious about for a long time. I wanted to see the letter of recommendation that Dr. Braun wrote for me when I was looking for a director's position. A copy was surely in the file of the hospital administration and at the HR department, and there was a chance I might be able to see it. In my first year as Director of Pathology, I did a good turn to the secretary in the administrative office of the hospital. Her husband had a biopsy of skin in a dermatologist's office and received a diagnosis of "early malignant melanoma", a potentially deadly tumor. The secretary, properly frightened, requested copies of the microscopic slides from the dermatologist and brought them to me for a review. I could not find any malignancy and thus forwarded the slides to Columbia University Hospital for an expert consultation. The consultant's diagnosis was "atypical nevus", and I had one of my little satisfactions. The secretary and her husband were overjoyed, as no further surgery or any other treatment was required. Atypical means "atypical", and it is just that.

One day, at lunch in the cafeteria, I sat next to the administrative secretary, and after chatting for a while, I dared to ask if she would let me have a peek at the letters of recommendation in my file. She looked at me for a moment and said:
"You know…, I really shouldn't do that! But…, I owe you a big one! Tomorrow, I'll let you have a quick look!"

The next day, she made copies and let me have them. I took them home to read them in the evening, in peace, after the children were put to bed.

Dr. Braun's letter was a full page, and at a quick first glance, it looked very good and sounded very positive. Reading again slowly, I noticed that one of my attributes was described more than once, and in a very emphatic manner. Apparently, I possessed "a deep sense for truth, always and in every instance," and then, in the next paragraph, I was described as "always completely candid" and later again as "positively truthful, without exception". This strong penchant for truth was obviously expressed with a purpose, so the reader would not miss my wonderful insistence on always telling the truth, even when it might not be completely appropriate. In a letter of recommendation, this was nothing but a backhanded slap. For a manager, a character of this kind could present trouble, a person not fit to be hired into the executive ranks. We all know how mighty inconvenient the truth can be on some occasions, and especially to certain people. Even though during all those years with Dr. Braun I had been particularly careful never to make an adverse comment on his work or ideas, in the end, he seemed to have a sense of what I felt. With his letter of recommendation, he just vented his feelings about one more of "those clowns".

As for ECOG, Dr. Braun never came back to any of its meetings. He must have been quite offended by the trick the ECOG principals played on him. I continued to work and participate in clinical research, collaborating with members of ECOG. Over the next 15 years, our pathology section published several practical papers about breast cancer and malignant tumors of bone and connective tissues.

Related to the active oncology program in the hospital, I regularly attended the weekly 'tumor board' meetings with surgeons, oncologists, radiotherapists, and radiologists, where every patient with a cancer diagnosis was presented and reviewed. The review included a discussion of clinical and X-ray findings, pathologic diagnosis, and finally, the plan for an appropriate protocol of therapy. These meetings were usually followed by a luncheon in the doctor's private dining room, with a continued discussion of medical cases.

At the time, the medical literature was replete with research articles showing that some of the special lymphocytes (white blood cells) had an important role in immunity, with suggestions that these little cells had an important function in the fight against cancer. During one of those lunches, I proposed, only in jest, but with a straight face, that it would be appropriate to ask the hospital chef to include in our tumor board lunch menu some sweetbreads. This was known to be a meal particularly rich in lymphocytes, and I said, it "might protect us all from cancer". After all, we were in an oncologic center. Soon thereafter, I was approached by the hospital cook, asking for a recipe for sweetbreads. It was the Medical Director, Dr. Blusher, who reacted to my proposal, and went to request from the cook the special 'oncologic' menu.

A large box of sweetbreads, the cook said, had already been waiting in the kitchen freezer. At home, Miriam had both the Larousse and Julia Child cookbooks, and it was easy to find the recipes. Henceforth, the weekly oncology luncheon included a platter of hot sweetbreads, a delicacy which was admittedly somewhat unhealthy for the arteries and was of doubtful value in cancer prevention. Nevertheless, the physicians enjoyed the new item on the menu, even if they did not believe it had any effect on cancer. Another lesson learned: making jokes with a straight face may lead to unexpected results.

Within the first several years in the hospital, I periodically uncovered in the records of the pathology department some of the old "Mickey Mouse" diagnoses, those first mentioned by Dr. Konig. Whenever a patient had surgery, it was customary to look up all previous records and diagnoses, together with a review of pertinent microscopic slides. There I encountered a few cases of malignant tumors that, upon review, were not at all malignant. Those cases were scattered over a spectrum of different organs and tissues, and each time it happened, it presented a delicate situation. I would verbally report it to the attending physician, usually a surgeon, and it was their business how to handle it with the patient... For me, it was nice to know that one more patient was free of a malignant tumor and could lead a normal life, free of cancer fear.

One day, my friend, Dr. Laporta came to ask for a favor. He was scheduled to make a presentation at the annual meeting of thoracic surgeons, where he would demonstrate one of his patients, who was successfully cured of lung cancer. At that point, the patient was 29 years old and completely free of tumor. Five years earlier, he received a diagnosis of cancer of the lung, a very rare occurrence at such a young age. For his presentation, Dr. Laporta needed pictures for projection, to demonstrate the microscopic appearance of the tumor. Of course, I would be glad to help. I had the microscopic slides pulled out of the old file, and reviewing them, I could not find any cancer. There was an uncommon benign tumor that sometimes arises in the lung. To be sure, I mailed copies of the microscopic slides for a formal consultation at Columbia University Hospital. Within ten days, I had a letter confirming the diagnosis of a benign tumor, an adenoma. I then called up Dr. Laporta and told him about the true nature of the tumor. He immediately came to see me, and when I showed him the letter of consultation, he was quite perplexed. He showed me a copy of the program for the annual meeting of thoracic surgeons, with the title of his presentation: "Cure of lung cancer in a 24-year-old man". He said that there was already a printed program for the meeting, and there was no time to change it. I told him there would be no problem...

I suggested a simple solution, so that the printed program could remain as it was. For his presentation, I would provide him with microscopic images of the tumor, and I advised him to first present the photographs without telling the audience the new diagnosis.

Seeing the projected microscopic images, the surgeons would not know the difference. Next, he should present to the audience exactly what happened. Before the case presentation, another pathologist reviewed the microscopic slides and made a diagnosis of a benign tumor, which was confirmed by the head of surgical pathology at Columbia University. I gave him a copy of the consultation. Finally, he could give the 'moral' of the story: 'When you get a diagnosis of cancer of lung in a 24-year-old man, it is best to ask for a second opinion, but from another pathology department'. And I let Dr. Laporta know about the concept of 'Mickey Mouse' diagnosis.

After returning from his meeting, Dr. Laporta came to thank me; his presentation was received very well. And in gratitude, he told me to come to his house and pick up a whole dressed deer. He was a hunter, and as he was a widower, he preferred to be invited for a good dinner. Henceforth, every year, during the hunting season, I received a whole deer, and I learned how to hang it out for a week and then skin it and carve out and freeze the best cuts.

We had an interesting Chairman of Obstetrics and Gynecology, Dr. Maguire, who did all his baby deliveries at our hospital. In two years, I received from him many dozens of placentas, but very rarely the tissue from a gynecologic procedure. One day at lunch, I asked him why he didn't do some more gynecologic work at our hospital. We were sitting together with other physicians, and I noticed that one of them, Dr. Konig, quietly chuckled. Dr. Maguire explained that his work was mostly concentrated on obstetrics. The next time I saw Dr. Konig, I asked him what he was chuckling about.

"Don't you know? Maguire does a lot of gynecologic surgery, some of it at the hospital in the neighboring town, where no one asks any questions, but most of it he does right in his private office."

"Hm, but he is our Chairman of OB-GYN?"

"Yes, and he has the largest gynecologic private practice in town!"

"Wow, I would never have thought…"

"Well, here, at this hospital, they better not know about it…"

"I guess there is no end to surprises."

"Yeah, you still have a few things to learn!"

But a couple of years later, somehow, it all came out into the open, and our Chairman of OB-GYN was called into the head administrator's office for a little discussion… I don't know what they talked about, but soon thereafter came an official hospital proclamation that our OB-GYN Chairman promised to forever cease doing any 'procedures' in his office. That made a big change: whatever followed was done much more discreetly.

It was in the early eighties that I started being interested in computers, and especially in their possible application in anatomic pathology and in clinical laboratory. I read a few books about laboratory computerization and about applying computers to keep a database of diagnostic reports. At the same time, I read about the first personal computers, and I bought the one made by Apple, the 5e model with little "floppy disks". Our children played with it, making pretty geometric designs, and I learned to program in a simple language called "basic". I felt it was time that my pathology office produces a streamlined output of pathologic diagnoses, with a database software for keeping records. The hospital provided my office with word processors, and on my own, I purchased a database software from

CAP (College of American Pathologists). It cost 500 dollars, and it contained a complete nomenclature of pathologic diagnoses. I loaded the database software into a word processor, and I had a quasi 'computerized' pathology office. Going forward, our look-up of previous records and diagnoses on each patient would be done with lightning speed, and I would no longer have to ask a secretary, to go and dig into a drawer with dusty old paper files.

At the same time, I proposed the computerization of the clinical lab, but since that would be a big and costly project, I had to wait for a decision from the group's central purchasing administration. When asked for an input, I provided the name of a company in Arizona that, according to my information, provided the most efficient lab software and hardware. However, the central purchasing mavens decided to purchase a computer system from another company. That required a whole year to first build a special room with a cooled double floor, and when the hardware was installed and became operational, it turned out to be tedious to run and labor-intensive to maintain. It was serviced by our in-house engineers, and it was frequently "down" for hours. After several years of struggling with that system, the hospital decided to look for a new lab computer, and then they chose the one from Arizona, which they originally rejected. By then, I was about to resign and leave for another position.

Chapter 12

Other Events and Observations

Aside from processing tissue biopsies, cytology and cell smears, blood, urine and other fluids, the Department of Pathology and Laboratory is also responsible for autopsies. An autopsy is done to determine and formally report the cause of death, and it is usually requested by the patient's next of kin, who must sign a permission. If the autopsy is requested or mandated by law, then the family's permission is not required. In that case, the pathologist acts as a coroner, and the autopsy report goes to the organ of law that ordered the autopsy. As director of pathology, I performed and supervised several coroner's cases, but one of them sticks to my memory, and it is worth recounting.

One day, the local police ambulance brought to the hospital the body of a one-year-old baby found dead at home in his crib. The police felt that it was most likely a case of a "sudden crib death", one of those rare and unexplained deaths that occur in infants. Nevertheless, they wanted an autopsy to ascertain that there was no other cause of death. My assistant pathologist went to perform the autopsy, and she found every organ in the body in normal condition. However, upon opening the skull, she found on the surface of the brain a few drops of fresh blood. She immediately called me to review her findings, and I saw that the blood looked fresh.

At that point, I took over the case and searched for the source of the blood. I examined the skull bone in the area corresponding to the position of blood on the brain surface, and there was a one inch long extremely thin straight line on the bone surface, representing a "hairline fracture". This was clearly the source of the blood. The corresponding outer side of the skull bone appeared smooth and intact. Then I carefully reviewed the skin of the scalp and found, hidden below the fine baby hair, a small, barely noticeable pink area of abrasion, again corresponding to the area of the hairline fracture inside the skull. The infant did not die of natural causes but of trauma to the head. It was a case where the law required an official legal medical investigation, with an autopsy done by a certified Medical Examiner. The infant's remains were wrapped in plastic and saved in the morgue refrigerator.

I contacted the office of the State Medical Examiner, described the preliminary autopsy findings, and asked for immediate intervention, to complete the autopsy. The Medical Examiner arrived in the late afternoon of the next day, stayed overnight in a hotel, and the following morning completed the autopsy. He took lots of photographs to document his findings, and before leaving, he unofficially confirmed the finding of a skull fracture, indicating that the cause of death was trauma to the head. His final written report would arrive in about one week and would be addressed directly to police authorities and the court. I was no longer responsible for the case but followed it as the story slowly unfolded over the next several months in the local press. Here is a summary of that sad story.

The infant died while under the care of a male babysitter, the boyfriend of the mother. The mother was working in a bar, and when she came home, she found the baby lying in the crib completely unresponsive, dead. The boyfriend claimed that he did not hear or know anything that could have caused the baby's death. The mother immediately informed the police, who came to the apartment with a legal search warrant. The detectives searched for any clues of foul play but did not find anything of interest. The boyfriend was sharply questioned, and he then remembered that at one point the baby cried, and he lifted him out of the crib "to calm him down" and then put him back into the crib, and the baby went to sleep.

Two weeks after the autopsy, I read in the local press that the Medical Examiner's office reported the cause of death as "trauma with fracture of the skull and cerebral damage". The case was referred to the court as a possible homicide. The prosecutor requested that detectives go back to the apartment and do a thorough second search for any physical clues of foul play. This time, the detectives found on the wall, right above the baby's crib, some faint pink stains with two baby hairs, and they took samples for examination. The stains contained, aside from baby hair, plasma fluid with a few blood cells that were identified as belonging to the baby. The babysitter was arrested and accused of having hit the baby's head against the wall. The case was declared a manslaughter.

Further along, the press reported that the defendant was on parole, out of jail after a felony, the nature of which was not revealed. The courts are always overloaded, and it took several months before the press reported that a court process had been scheduled. The defendant's attorney was provided by his uncle, a powerful local politician. During the court proceedings, the attorney's main goal was to bar the police from showing any findings or evidence from the second search of the apartment. The catch was that the police failed to obtain a new search warrant for the repeat examination of the apartment. The evidence of the defendant's complicity in the infant's death was thereby suppressed on a technicality. During intense interrogation by the prosecutor, the defendant remembered that the baby was crying very hard, and to calm him down, he "lifted him up and shook him a few times" ... The outcome of the court process was that the defendant walked out free and continued to serve his parole time.

* * *

I practiced in a town with a sizable medical community that provided some interesting observations. There was a large group of orthopedic surgeons practicing under the leadership of Dr. O'Grady, chairman of the orthopedics department in our hospital. He owned an entire office building, with multiple individual doctor's offices, X-ray equipment, and facilities for rehabilitation therapy. Located in an area with long winters and lots of ice and snow, the main business of the orthopedic surgeons in winter was to deal with trauma and fractures. As a pathologist, I received lots of metallic prostheses from broken hips, those that failed and had to be replaced. One brand was particularly prone to failure due to the shedding of metallic particles into the surrounding tissues, with attendant displacement, pain and black discoloration of adjacent ligaments. That brand was eventually pulled off the market, and I wondered how it was possible that it was ever approved for use.

Another large part of the orthopedic practice in summer was devoted to the treatment of painful knees. The common treatment at that time consisted of arthroscopy, with the shaving of the damaged (cracked) cartilage surfaces inside the knee joint. When I developed pain in both knees after playing tennis on hard courts, our orthopedists immediately offered to cure me by means of arthroscopy. Having spent a lot of time studying bone and cartilage pathology in an orthopedic hospital, I thanked them and declined the arthroscopic treatment.

The knee pain following jogging or running is caused by small cracks in the surface of the cartilage. Shaving off the cracked surface by arthroscopy requires a longer recovery time than if one just stops all athletic activity and gives the joints a few months of rest. One ought to know that the cartilage, just like the fingernails, continues to grow during our entire life. The surface of the cartilage slowly sheds its top layer of cells into the fluid of the joint space, where it is digested by the synovial cells of the joint capsule. The shedding of the top cell layer lets the underlying cartilage move upward and create a new, smooth surface. Thus, the cracks "grow out" and disappear, and the joint becomes free of pain. This process takes several months, but it is still a far better choice than arthroscopic surgery. My pain started in June, and in November, by the time we had good snow, I was able to enjoy downhill skiing without any pain.

Knee arthroscopy was a treatment of choice for several decades, even though the recovery after surgery took more time than if one were treated by resting, not to count the cost of the treatment. It was only quite recently, in 2015, that articles finally started appearing in medical literature, clearly stating that arthroscopic knee surgery does more harm than good. Here is a reference: "Arthroscopic Surgery for Degenerative Knee: Systematic Review and Meta-analysis of Benefits and Harms," JB Thorlund, CB Juhl, EM Roos, LM Lohmander; BMJ: June 2015, with a review by: DG Fairchild, MD, MPH and L Di Francesco, MD, MPH, FACP, FHM, who conclude with the following statement: "Available evidence supports the reversal of a common medical practice".

Even before the above revelations, it was reported that about 70 orthopedic surgeons moved out of California, mostly from San Diego and other warm, dry weather areas. Most of them moved into the upper Midwest, where there was a shortage of orthopedic services. The joggers of California finally found out that they no longer needed their painful knees treated by arthroscopy.

One winter, our eight-year-old daughter fell on ice and broke her clavicle. Miriam took her to Dr. O'Grady's office. X-rays were taken, and I was informed that the bone was well aligned, and with a proper cast, it would heal within about three weeks. As expected, when the cast was taken off, a second X-ray showed perfect healing. I thanked Dr. O'Grady for his care, and very soon, we all forgot about the fracture. About two months after the accident, I received in the mail copies of payments made by our insurance company.

Upon review of the charges, I was glad to see that everything was fully paid. It only struck me as odd that, according to the charges, our daughter had visited and was examined in Dr. O'Grady's office four times. When I asked Miriam about it, she was positive that she visited that office only twice: the first time immediately after the accident, and the second time, when the cast was taken off. No doubt, the charges for two additional visits were a clerical error. I did not think it was appropriate to call and bother Dr. O'Grady about a little clerical mistake made accidentally by his staff.

A few months later, a young orthopedic surgeon, who had only recently joined Dr. O'Grady's group practice, one day came to inform me that he had separated from the group practice and that I should send all pathologic reports of his patients to his new office address. I was surprised and remarked that it might be hard for him to practice all by himself. He told me that he had to leave the group practice because he did not agree with the way his patients were handled by the office staff. His explanation was somewhat cryptic, but I did not dwell on it.

A few months later, I read in the news that overnight, there was a big fire in town involving a building on a principal street. It was Dr. O'Grady's office building, and unfortunately, it burned down to the ground before the firemen could save it. The cause of the fire was never found, but luckily, the office building was well-insured. It was only a shame, the press reported, that all patients' records were completely lost...

In the special environment of a small town, I encountered for the first time a few physicians whose medical offices functioned in the perfect style of a "small business". There was a Dr. Johnson, the internist, who had in the waiting room a large sign: "CASH ONLY", and it meant up front. Then there was a Dr. Hamid, a young cardiologist, who opened a large private office which soon became so busy that he had no time to ever take his specialty Board examination. Within two years, he was reported in the news as having done the largest number of cardiac catheterizations in the North-East. People wondered if this achievement would be placed into the Guinness Book of records. It seemed, whoever walked into this cardiologist's office, received a cardiac catheterization. After his record was published in the press, the annual number of catheterizations at his office in the subsequent years became somewhat reduced...

A highly recommended dentist in town, Dr. Guilder, found on my very first check-up a "bad tooth". It was a wisdom tooth, a third molar in the lower jaw, barely protruding out of the gum. Dr. Guilder diagnosed it as having "caries", a decay. Since it was a wisdom tooth and did not seem functional, Dr. Guilder felt it would be best to remove it. I tried to protest:

"But I have no pain, and in over 40 years, it never bothered me!"

"It is a bad, decayed tooth! It should come out, or you will have trouble with it later!"

"Well then..." - I gave in to the strong assurance, and he proceeded to numb my gum, and after a few minutes took a hold of the tooth and started pulling on it. He pulled so hard that droplets of sweat appeared on his forehead. The tooth would not budge. With numbed lips, I mumbled:

"Aare you shiur, zis toof is bad?"

"Defin'ly. I've no doubt!" and he picked up a heavier, larger pair of pliers and dug into my gum to get a better grip. He again started pulling with all his might, sweat pouring down his brow. Dr. Guilder was a big man and quite portly, and he pulled on my tooth so hard that he began to lift me out of the chair. He moaned and gave one heavier yank on the tooth, and suddenly, with a big thud, he fell backward onto the floor. For a few moments, he was stunned and remained sitting on his fat ass. The pliers slipped out of his hand, and my tooth rolled away towards the corner of the room. While Dr. Guilder was trying to get back on his feet, I jumped out of the chair, picked up the tooth, and put it in my pocket. I had not seen in a long time what a tooth decay looked like under the microscope, and I wanted to have a look at its pathology. One week later, the tooth was well decalcified and soft, and I got nicely stained sections of it under my microscope. It appeared perfectly normal, just like in those pictures in the books of normal anatomy. No decay of any kind could be seen. I sent Dr. Guilder the pathologic report: "Normal third molar tooth" accompanied with a separate short note, indicating that the report was gratis. Then I inquired around and found a decent dentist, one with whom my whole family stayed for the next twelve years.

Also established in town was a Dr. Trucker, an ENT specialist who recently graduated from medical school and residency training, with the help of an Army tuition for his good service in Vietnam. Whenever I tried to call him about an important finding on one of his patients, his telephone would be answered by a recorded message: "Please listen for the following sound..." and I would listen and hear nothing but a deep silence... Then the voice would continue: "...now, if you did not hear any sound, you may need a hearing aid. Please make an appointment for a free hearing test." Only after that message would I finally hear a live secretary, "Hello? How may I help…"

Dr. Trucker was not only seeing patients, but his office was also in the business of testing the hearing and selling hearing aids. It could be that he was trying to recover from the fact that the lucrative mass removals of tonsils and adenoids in children were finally declared unnecessary and unwarranted.

What then became popular among some of the ENT specialists was a new procedure: insertion of a tiny plastic tube into the eardrum of every child who had an ear inflammation, a condition that nearly every child gets at least 3 to 4 times in life. As a pathologist, over the years, I received thousands of specimens with little plastic ear tubes because they had to be eventually removed, which required one more procedure. Several years later, the ear tube treatments would also be found unnecessary, and they were largely discontinued.

As recounted by a nurse from the operating room, that same Dr. Trucker, on one occasion inserted an ear tube into the wrong ear, the healthy one. He took it in stride, turned the child around, and presto, inserted another ear tube into the opposite ear, which was inflamed. Then he explained to the parents that "as a precaution," he put the tubes in *both* ears, but would charge them for only one…

In the early eighties, when the first reports appeared describing an odd illness in gay men in San Francisco, I did not think much about it and hoped that it would soon go away and be forgotten. I was wrong: within a couple of years, it became clear that the odd new disease was caused by a virus, the Human Immunodeficiency Virus (HIV), and the illness caused by it was called Acute Immune Deficiency Syndrome (AIDS). It was subsequently found to be highly infectious and transmitted by personal contact through blood or body fluids, and it was present all around the world, spreading both in men and women, mostly by sexual contact (STD) or by drug use with contaminated needles. In 1983 scientists throughout the US and Western Europe recommended that blood banks refuse donations of blood from persons who had a history of possible contact with HIV-infected individuals. As Director of Pathology and Laboratory, I was responsible for blood bank compatibility testing and the safety of all blood and blood components for transfusion. *

One day, in the mid-eighties, the local court asked me to give a deposition regarding a lawsuit against the hospital. The lawsuit was brought by a 19-year-old woman who, while applying for a marriage license, had a shocking discovery that she was HIV positive. It was objectively ascertained that she did not acquire the HIV through sexual activity, but a year earlier, when she had surgery and received a transfusion of one unit of blood. I was provided with the name of the patient, and indeed, the records showed that the lab issued a unit of blood for transfusion, apparently for anemia. When I looked at the date of the blood transfusion, it appeared that it was given a few months before our government ordered that all blood products for transfusion must be tested and confirmed as negative for HIV. It was most unfortunate that more than one year passed since the time when the scientists recommended that blood collection centers take steps to not accept blood from donors who might be infected with HIV, till a test for HIV became available, and the government ordered that all blood donors must be tested for HIV.

---

*A reliable test for HIV became available in the beginning of 1985, and by the end of April of that year the blood collection centers in US began to test all blood donors. By end of July 1985, the blood supply in US was declared free of AIDS virus.

During that unfortunate period, uncounted recipients of transfusions were infected with HIV, and one well known victim was the tennis player Artur Ashe. As reported in the press, a considerably longer delay in blood testing for HIV occurred in Switzerland and in France, where many people were unnecessarily infected. Similar statistics from certain countries of Eastern Europe and Asia do not exist because in those countries HIV had been declared as non-existent - until many years later.

The delay in recognizing HIV as a threat to the entire human race was in great part caused by politicians together with a segment of the society that refused to be concerned with an illness which supposedly involved only people who were being shunned and considered 'abnormal'. To my knowledge, of all the government officials responsible for undue delays in HIV testing of blood donors to prevent AIDS, only one person, a secretary of health in France was convicted on account of his poor decision, and he ended up with a very short jail sentence.

When I gave the court deposition regarding our hospital lawsuit, I clearly stated that the infection in the 19-year-old girl occurred before all blood products were ordered to be tested for HIV. Two months after the deposition, I was informed that I would have to give another deposition for the same case. When I inquired about the reason for the repeat deposition, I was told that "the original record was lost". During the second deposition I made the same statement about the reason for the infection. That time, I added that the lawsuit against the hospital should be either dismissed or redirected towards those who, despite scientists' recommendations, did not follow steps to prevent acceptance of blood from donors at risk for HIV infection. The lawsuit against the hospital was eventually dismissed.

After I was in town for a couple of years, the news slowly spread that there was a pathologist with a special interest in cancer diagnosis, particularly of breast and bone tumors. Some private consultations began to trickle my way from other regional hospitals and doctor's offices. Those consultations were a sign that my work in the area was being recognized.

One day, I received a phone call from a pathologist who was the vice president of a medical laboratory company in Canada, and he asked me whether I would be interested in the position of "consultant pathologist". The Canadian company owned multiple small satellite clinical laboratories in the entire North-East of the US, and it needed a consultant specifically to organize the handling of biopsies and to develop procedures for managing cytology. I had to first check with my hospital administration, and since the consultant position was not in conflict with the hospital, it was approved. I accepted the job.

The Canadian company was receiving a very large volume of PAP smears and, at the same time it filed for a patent on a computerized PAP screening device that would eliminate the need for hiring cytology screeners. I found the work interesting; the job did not require too much of my time, and it carried a decent remuneration, which would supplement the very small annual salary raises during a period of high inflation. A little extra income would be of help towards our children's college tuitions.

As a consultant, I attended quarterly meetings in Toronto, usually held over a weekend, and this did not interfere with my hospital job. Once a year, the Canadian company organized a major management course for all consultants and directors of the satellite labs. This course always put a great emphasis on "leadership", and the main theme would feature a well-known person, a "real leader". Once it was about the leader of a successful expedition that conquered the summit of Mt.

Everest: another time, it was about Alexander the Great, and yet another time, it was about Napoleon; all of them were considered "great leaders". Each time, the course would repeatedly emphasize that "a leader is born", meaning that a leader carries in his or her genetic makeup a talent, having a rare and special gift to lead and manage people. On the other hand, the course lecturer told us that all of us should try to learn the principles of management so that we become better leaders in our current positions.

It was a little hard to understand how one could "learn" to be a leader, while we were told that "a leader is born" with an inherent "talent" or a "gift" of genetic origin. There seemed to be some contradiction in terms. To be the head of an organization requires, first, common sense, and then some experience in dealing with people and directing them. Ever since childhood, I acquired a personal idiosyncrasy for the word "leader". It is because the first language I spoke was German. The word "leader" in German is "Führer", and "Der Führer" was a notorious "leader" responsible for the murder of millions of people, a name that resonates in my mind with horror and evil.

I enjoyed working as a consultant with the Canadian company and became friendly with several principals of that firm, but there was an issue in the culture of that company that rubbed me the wrong way. It was the principal theme of their management courses, a theme that idolized historic persons, "leaders" like Alexander the Great and Napoleon. These two army generals were great military strategists, but their "success" was responsible for violent deaths of hundreds of thousands of people. Theirs was a leadership marked by brute force, war, and conquest with subjugation of others, and I could not see anything admirable in that sort of leadership.

Reasonable people can work together, even if they do not subscribe to the same doctrine, religion, culture, or philosophy. People and cultures do change, and there is always hope that with time, people may acquire new, better ideas. I remained a consultant with the Canadian firm for over ten years till the time I relocated to another part of the country. What is left from that relationship are good memories of personal friendships and good times with a few people in Toronto and a little gold pin received for ten years of service.

After years of serving as Director of Pathology and Laboratory in a rural area, I began actively seeking a similar position in a location closer to large urban center. Both Miriam and I really preferred to live closer to a place with easier access to cultural events, theaters, museums, etc., something that was sorely lacking locally. Another reason for wanting to relocate was that two of our children were already away at college, and the other two were soon to be done with high school. We also wanted to move closer to some of our old friends from the sixties and seventies, people who we knew from the time when we started raising a family, friends with whom we continued to be in touch throughout the eighties.

At the same time, looking at what happened in the area where we lived, we saw a slow, steady decline. Most of the large industries either pulled out and moved to other parts of the country, or they were bought out and dismantled, or they went bankrupt. We lived in the "rust belt". The largest company in the area decreased from over 10,000 employees down to about 2,000. The value of the local real estate was going down.

The only local business that was growing larger was the scrap yard. It belonged to one of the wealthiest men in town, a man nicknamed "Paper Tiger". He collected everything that was discarded, but most of all, paper and scrap metal, which he sold to be recycled. With respect to recycling, he was prescient! He got rich dealing with scrap, way before it became popular to recycle metal and paper throughout the country. He was also known as a "poet". A little strophe of his, under a rubric "Paper Tiger" would regularly appear in the local press. It was a good advertisement for getting all the scrap into his yard.

Speaking about Mister Paper Tiger, here is an episode that happened not long after Miriam and I came to live in that town, and it could be said that Paper Tiger helped us to quickly meet and get to know a lot of people. We met him in person only once at a lavish charity dinner given in his honor.

That famous dinner party was attended by local college professors, lawyers, accountants, physicians, engineers, business owners, people of cloth (of all kinds), and most of the "who is who" personalities in the area, naturally, including the wives or partners. All in all, there were about 250 guests. The affair was festive, with formal evening attire, and it was catered in a very spacious venue. There were round tables, large enough to seat ten people, all set with linen tablecloths, fine porcelain dishes, ornate silverware wrapped in a fine cloth napkin, and fine glassware, three per setting, fancy salt and pepper shakers, condiments, bottled water, and a vase with beautiful flowers in the center of each table. At first, as usual, the affair started with cocktails and canapés and soft drinks, people standing in little groups or mingling and cruising around, showing their attire and their faces, meeting everybody and busily chatting, mostly about nothing. Then, it was announced that the speaker for the evening would be the Paper Tiger and that he would give a speech in the form of a poem. We were asked to sit at our designated tables, and we found ours, fortunately somewhat towards the corner of the room and distant from the speaker's podium.

We were seated together with people of our choice, an attorney, an older college professor, and two physicians, all with their wives, and all of whom we had known quite well. At the neighboring tables sat many couples who we also knew. Silence was requested and Paper Tiger began to read, or rather, to declaim his poem. It was an ode to various worthy citizens and institutions, somewhat epic in length, and delivered in a Shakespearian style, if not by content, then by intent. There came long, Latin-sounding expressions and some newly made-up words, like "fermentated", which was rhymed with "lubricated", and all was spiced with a wide poetic freedom.

Even though Miriam and I happened to sit with our backs to the speaker's podium, we could clearly hear every elocution and syllable. Large black speaker boxes were strategically positioned in all corners of the room, and one of them, close to our table, delivered the blather straight to our faces.

As the Paper Tiger went on at some length, I started throwing occasional sideways glances to my right, at Miriam, and I caught her too, now and then, throwing me a knowing look. At that point, not to lose concentration on the precious content of the poem, I thought it was best to look down at my empty plate or at the flowers straight in front of me, and just listen to the lilting stream of words, steadily quavering from the speaker box:

"…and such a fair… and pleasant… intercourse… with all our stupendous… citizens…, 'bout our prodigious… carriers of esteem… and consequence…", and on it went.

Overcome by an unstoppable urge to laugh, I kept my mouth open and the larynx well relaxed, so that my breath could go in and out without making any sound, while my belly muscles were producing spasms of laughter that shook my whole body. A quick side glance at Miriam let me know that she, too, had caught it; it was contagious. She saw me, and we both were silently shaking in our chairs with spasms of soundless laughter, heads down, looking into the empty porcelain plates in front. To help suppress the spasms, I held my forearms firmly across the stomach. Then I saw Miriam lean forward and steady herself by placing both forearms against the edge of the table. The round wooden tabletop, apparently sitting on a central base and stabilized merely by its massive weight, suddenly started to vibrate, ever so slightly echoing the silent shivers of Miriam's laughter. The three empty glasses, placed close to one another, started making clicking, jangling noises, on and on, going all around the table… I peeped around and saw the old college professor on my left raise his right hand up behind the ear and fiddle with his fingers. Well, I thought, *he just turned off his hearing aid!*

Then the soft jangling noises began coming from a few neighboring tables. The Paper Tiger, far away, up on the podium, was oblivious and completely engrossed and enthralled by his poem. He kept declaiming, and we, no longer listening, directed all our strength and power to stop the damn laughter. And we somehow did succeed. Then soon, the speaker box fell silent, everybody stood up, and there was the usual loud applause. Finally, we sat down, our faces still red from laughter. After a while, the waiters removed our empty plates, and the fancy dinner service, soup and wine and all, began for real.

Somebody from our table must have spoken, because after that evening, we became not exactly celebrities, but well known in town. Everyone knew who started the jangling of the glassware. In the following weeks, most people we knew began to approach us with a friendly smile, and then happily reminisce about the festive evening dinner… It's true; we heard that a few people appeared indignant.

The charity dinner was a success: at the end of dinner service, when the pledge call came around, we all opened our purses, and, guilty as we were, gave away more money than was expected. A new sports facility for the children would be built soon thereafter. We all agreed that the Paper Tiger should be praised! He was the Man of the town, and his zeal to recirculate every scrap was truly uplifting our spirits.

Over all those years when I worked, I always felt good practicing my profession and, despite occasional problems, I liked my job to a point where I never counted the hours. In fact, I put in lots of overtime voluntarily and without regret. One might consider me a workaholic, but I simply did not feel that way, because the bulk of routine work was done fast and with ease, while the harder diagnostic cases gave me the pleasure of that certain excitement which comes with solving problems.

It is true that in my career I spent a lot of hours working, often more than one job, but it is also true that I took time off for sport and recreation, and every year I utilized all vacation time I was allowed. "Work hard and play hard!" Aided by the climate in the North-East, I enjoyed plenty of skiing in the icy local mountains. That practice served me well when I turned 50 and became eligible for the NASTAR 'senior' handicap. Competing in slalom, I received a silver and two bronze medals.

My annual summer vacation was spent either together with family, or every second year our children were placed into a summer camp, while Miriam and I took time to travel. Our destination was usually Western Europe, mostly Italy, France and Switzerland, where, over the years we collected some priceless memories. Living in the North-East, the long winters compelled us to regularly take a week's break on a Caribbean island. We especially liked Aruba, Bonaire, the Grenadines and Guadeloupe and Martinique. The two French islands had Club Med resorts which were reasonably priced and offered many types of sport recreation, including even sailing with an instructor, but without additional charges. This brings me to a little episode on a flight to a Club Med.

The Club organized charter flights, usually with a less well-known airline, using simple airplanes that seat six people in each row with an aisle in the middle, and the entire aircraft was just economy class with minimal cabin service. As we relaxed in our seats, about an hour into the flight, we noticed aside from the regular cigarette smoke an odd, unfamiliar odor. Then, there was a light tap on my shoulder from the passenger behind me who leaned forward into the aisle and quietly said:

"Hey! Enjoy and pass it on!" while handing me a lit cigarette. I realized it was a 'joint'! A little stunned, I held it in my hand and recognized the odd smell. I showed the joint to Miriam, we looked at each other, and then I said:

"Ladies first!" and offered it to the quiet young woman in the window seat next to us. She took it without hesitation, and after taking two short draws, handed it to Miriam, who held it like you hold a piece of dirt, and quickly passed it to me. I tapped the shoulder of the guy in front of me and passed it to him.

The young woman in the seat next to us looked at me and said:

"Don't you…?"

"No. We feel perfectly happy as we are…". *

Within the next half hour, the joints kept coming each which way, and we just passed them on. Meanwhile, the air in the cabin was getting more and more pungent. Suddenly, a loud announcement from the pa system gave a jolt to everyone around:

---

*Smoking on US domestic flights of less than 6 hours duration was banned only in 1990, and that took an act of Congress. Smoking on all domestic and international flights was banned in year 2000.

"Attention! ATTENTION! This is your captain speaking! Passengers, PLEASE, EXTINGUISH ALL CIGARETTES NOW! We are getting too much smoke on deck, in the cockpit! We need to be able to fly this aircraft! Thank you for your attention!"

After a long moment of silence, a light murmuring and whispering was heard throughout the cabin, and then there was just the droning noise of the jet engines. The air in the cabin soon became much lighter. As I looked around, the people's faces reflected a happy mood, many wearing a smile. Miriam and I sat through the rest of the flight and talked about the smooth warm sand, the blue water with colorful fish, and the ever-changing Caribbean sunsets that expected us at our destination…

* * *

When I hinted to some of my closest friends that I was thinking finding a new job closer to a large city, their reaction was plain discouraging. One of them said:

"Peter! Wake up! You are over fifty!" and another one:

"At your age, who'll give you a job?"

"Maybe somebody will!"

"But, why on Earth would you want to leave? Don't you like it here?"

"Because I've done all that could be done in my present position. And now I'd like to move on…"

That's what I would answer, and it was the truth, although it was only a part of the truth. The other reasons for wanting to leave, I could not tell them. It wouldn't be nice… Every now and then, the subject of my leaving town would again resurface, and one or another of my friends would begin to bug me:

"Are you still trying to find a job?"

"Maybe!"

"Well… Good luck!"

Then, another one would begin:

"But really, where could you go that's so much better? Why do you even want to leave?"

A little annoyed and only half joking, I would say:

"Because I don't want to die here!" with emphasis on "here". That was not nice, but it was true.

And then it happened! I did get a new position, and it was time to part. All our friends gave us a big party and gifts and souvenirs, and so did the people with whom I worked in the hospital. Twelve and a half years! I was happy to help the administration find a new director to replace me; it was a colleague from another local hospital about 30 miles away. Most of our friends remained in the area till they retired. Then, most also left, scattered, all in different directions, mostly to Florida or Arizona. Our pediatrician, fed up with his boring job of weighing and measuring the growth of healthy children, had moved away a year before us. He went to Philadelphia and took a job as a consultant for a large pharmaceutical company. I still remember the jubilation of his wife, when we came to say goodbye. She declared that she wanted only to enjoy the "brotherly love" of a real city. But there was one dear friend who remained steadfast and still resides in that little town where he was born and where he grew up. We continue to exchange cards and phone calls with him and his wife at least once a year.

Sadly, three years after we left town, we had to go back for a funeral. My dearest friend, Dr. Konig, had a sudden massive heart attack and died.

Several years later, after I retired and we moved to the West Coast, we heard that Dr. Konig's wife, while substituting for a teacher in the local high school, was shot and killed by an angry young man. She was asked to cover for another teacher, just for one single day, and she was murdered! It was a tragic accident that was hard to comprehend.

Chapter 13

The Job Search

In 42 years of medical practice, I experienced only a little more than a dozen job interviews. Each one of my last three positions was of long duration that lasted 8, 12.5 and 13.5 years. Most of my job interviews were short, easy and relaxed. If it was a good match, I would be called back for a second round, and after that, either I would receive a short letter, stating that another candidate was chosen, or I would receive a job offer, followed by a meeting and discussion about the salary and benefits.

In the 70s and 80s, many hospitals, particularly in larger cities, suffered heavy financial losses and had to be closed. The financial difficulties were partly due to very low reimbursement rates, tightly controlled by insurance carriers or by Medicare and Medicaid. The hospitals were also financially strapped by employing a full staff, while many beds were not occupied. One had to watch out, not to take a job in a hospital that might be closing within a year or two. A job interview was a two-way road. The issue of the hospital's future had to be delicately investigated, along with all other details about the position. Among all my job interviews, two were remarkable, and they have remained deeply etched in my memory.

When I decided to end my academic career and get a position of Director of Pathology and Laboratory in a community hospital, I found several hospital ads, none in NYC, but mostly in the suburban or relatively remote exurban areas, and I responded by sending my resume, waiting to be contacted. My very first interview for the position of Director of Pathology and Laboratory was in a suburban hospital, very close to NYC. The interview went very smoothly, but the hospital chose another candidate.

My next interview, at the end of February in 1977, was at a large suburban hospital located in a small town, about an hour from Philadelphia and about two hours from NYC, close to a major highway. The interview was held by the Medical Board, led by the Chairman of the Board and chief of surgery, Dr. Smith. He explained that the job opening was rather sudden, and it was a sort of emergency: both previous pathologists had recently been dismissed, and the reason was not given. The members of the board threw at me many questions, mostly related to their specialty, and I had no trouble answering them. Dr. Smith said, the board had at least one other candidate to interview, and I would hear about their decision within a week. Following the interview, a member of the board, an internist, took me on a tour of the Department of Pathology and Laboratory, and there I met a pathologist who was serving as a temporary "locum tenens". An important fact was that the hospital census was high, and there was a sufficient supply of patients throughout the year. I found that there was a sort of arrangement, whereby the hospital received all accident victims from a major highway that ran nearby. The hospital appeared safe from financial problems.

As it was customary, I contacted the previous two pathologists, to hear their opinion about the hospital and the job. I obtained their phone numbers, and when I called, both would not say why they left their job, but each one stated that the hospital administrator, Mr. Adams, was "difficult to work with". I liked the hospital, and felt that, if offered the position, I would be willing to take the risk and find out, just how difficult a man was that administrator.

About a week later, I was called for a second interview, again with the Medical Board, and it went very well. Three days later, I received a letter of appointment to the position of Director of Pathology and Laboratory, signed by the Chairman of the Medical Board, Dr. Smith. The letter also informed me that for the details of my remuneration and benefits package, I should set up a meeting with the administrator, Mr. Adams. I was happy and excited, but of course, did not want to tell anyone about the appointment before having a final discussion with the administrator and a signed contract.

The meeting with the administrator was scheduled for the first week of March 1977, on a Monday at 10 am. I arrived at the hospital in time for the meeting and was promptly ushered into Mr. Adams's office. He immediately started telling me about the hospital's long history and excellent reputation. Within about fifteen minutes, Mr. Adams received a phone call, and I was excused to wait in the secretary's office. Our meeting continued for nearly two hours, because there were four more phone interruptions, and each time, I was excused and had to wait outside for about ten minutes.

During most of the meeting, Mr. Adams talked at great length, either describing the advantages of the hospital, or explaining the details about the package of benefits. The benefits were very generous, especially the pension plan, and finally, Mr. Adams came out with my annual salary. It was surprisingly high: 90,000 dollars! That was at least 10,000 above the usual amount for a director's job in that region. The job required two full-time pathologists, and Mr. Adams proposed that I contact and engage the other candidate, the runner-up for the director's job. I did not like the idea; I would have preferred to hire an assistant pathologist of my own choice but having received such a generous salary offer, I agreed. Mr. Adams gave me a copy of the other candidate's resume with his phone number and address and said I should interview him as soon as possible. We parted with the understanding that within a couple of days I would receive in the mail a contract with a copy to be signed and returned to the hospital.

After the meeting with Mr. Adams, I sat in my car and first looked over the resume of the candidate I was to hire as Assistant Pathologist. He was from Philadelphia and had about the same years of experience as I, but he was trained and certified only in Anatomic Pathology and had no experience in clinical laboratory. This was somewhat reassuring, and I felt he would not present a threat to my job. It was surprising that he was even considered for directorship of the entire department. Upon returning home, I first gave the good news to Miriam, and the same afternoon, I called up the pathologist in Philadelphia, and we set up a date for our meeting next weekend at a mutually convenient location.

The next day in the evening Mr. Adams called me at home. After introducing himself, immediately after I greeted him, he said:

"Listen, I want to inform you of something important! We are continuing the search for a head pathologist!"

"Excuse me, can you, please, explain what—" but he cut me off, saying loud and clear:

"I am informing you that as of now, our search for a head pathologist is continuing! Have a good evening!", and he hung up.

I was stunned. His statement was quite clear, though, and no matter how incredible it sounded, I understood it very well. For some reason, I was being rejected from the job! Half in disbelief, I went on to read my letter of appointment, signed by the Chairman of the Medical Board. *How can this be?* I thought. That night, it was hard to fall asleep and harder yet, to stay asleep. I could not wait for the next morning to call Dr. Smith, the Chairman of the Medical Board, and find out what caused the sudden change.

Early next morning, when I made that call, his secretary took a message and said he was in surgery. I explained the urgency of my call, and she promised he would call me back as soon as he was free. I called the pathologist in Philadelphia and canceled our appointment. He did not ask any question, but informed me that the day before, he had been called by Mr. Adams to come in for a meeting with him! It seemed that Mr. Adams preferred to have a Director of Pathology who was not certified in clinical laboratory.

Later that morning, Dr. Smith returned my call. When I asked why Mr. Adams suddenly called me to say that the hospital was continuing the search for a head pathologist, he replied:

"Mr. Adams told me you demanded way too much money!" This was astounding, and I calmly said:

"I made no demand whatsoever! It was Mr. Adams who did most of the talking. He first explained to me the benefits package, and finally offered a salary of 90,000. I did not ask for anything! I only accepted what Mr. Adams offered and made no demand at all! Mr. Adams also suggested that I hire the runner-up candidate as an assistant pathologist and gave me his resume, asking that I meet with him to discuss our arrangem—", but Dr. Smith interrupted:

"Was there anyone else present during your meeting with Mr. Adams?"

"No, we were alone, in his office."

"Well, I will call you back in the afternoon. I must go back into surgery."

Late that afternoon, the busy surgeon called back, and he sounded upset and angry, and he said:

"Mr. Adams insists that you demanded too much money and benefits!"

"This is absolutely not true! Dr. Smith, please, believe me! I made no demands, none what-so-ever!"

"You know... I do believe you! But unfortunately, as there was no witness, I must take the word of the administrator! In the future, I will see to it that Mr. Adams negotiates with an appointee only in the presence of a member of the Medical Board. I am sorry, but at this point, I cannot do anything about it."

"Well, thank you for calling…Goodbye."

I was shocked by the administrator's blatant lies, but I realized, though it was hard to believe it, that an administrator could overrule the entire Medical Board.

I was very, very upset. To this day, I can hardly find the right words to describe the level of my disappointment, the sheer aggravation, the awful feeling of letdown, the weight of the deceit, the burden pressing on my mind. It was a bitter pill to swallow, and it made me think of what I learned from life: that there is no such thing as "fair", and that "equal" exists only in math…*

I could feel that Dr. Smith believed me and that he was disturbed and quite mad about the whole affair, because the administrator made an ass of him too. I knew it was no use getting aggravated, and I consoled

---

* In this instance, when I say "fair", I am merely referring to the concept of "fairness", the sense of what is just and honest and the right thing to do. In real life, everyone has his or her own idea of what is "fair", and thus, who is to say, what represents fairness or fair behavior?? Along the same line, it may be hard to find "equality" among humans…

myself that, fortunately I had not revealed to anyone that I received this "wonderful" appointment.

A day later, when I felt a little calmer, I called a close friend and told him all the details, exactly as it happened. He listened very intently and then gave me his advice:

"You can take a good lawyer and sue the hospital and the Medical Board Chairman for a breach of contract. You have a signed letter of appointment, and you could get a compensation of at least one year's salary, and maybe you could get even more for all the pain and aggravation. Of course, nearly half the money would go for the lawyer's fee, but still, you would have the satisfaction of…", but I was no longer listening to him. My mind had already begun to churn my own thoughts.

As soon as my friend took a breath, and for a split second stopped talking, I interrupted him, and poured it out:

"Well, thanks for the advice! But the way I feel right now…, to sue and start with lawyers, I really don't like it! It's not my way, especially not, while I am still looking for a job. First, I don't want to have a lawsuit on my record! Second, a litigation would be aggravating and distasteful, and it may last for months or even years, only to poison my mind! I will try, only try, to forget all of this! Thanks for listening! By offering me advice, you helped me to move on! I just must forget and move on! Thanks!"

"You are welcome. And try to calm down!"

"Good advice! Bye."

Then, I began to think about what to do next. In the following days, I called all my colleagues and friends and looked at all the advertisements, trying to find an open position for a Director of

Pathology and Laboratory. Though meanwhile, I felt constant aggravation! And how it lasted! For the next three weeks, I was so much beside myself that I just could not sleep. Every night, I turned and turned again in my bed and slept no more than a total of two hours. The rest of the night, I lay and just kept changing positions, turning this way and that way. I kept thinking and raking my brains about what happened and why it happened. The question gnawed at me. *Why? But why?* I regurgitated the entire conversation with Mr. Adams... Was it because, when he asked me whether I had spoken to the two previous pathologists, I truthfully answered that I had just followed the protocol of the College of American Pathologists. I told him, it was a brief call, just asking for any useful information about the job, and each one of them gave me a brief positive comment, ending the call in about 2-3 minutes. *Perhaps Mr. Adams didn't like the mere fact that I called the pathologists? He must have had a reason to reject me, but I would never know what it was... Maybe he did not like my resume or my whole background? In any case, he preferred the other, less qualified candidate.*

Little by little, I let go of all those useless thoughts. Only the passage of time could bring me healing! And what would help, most of all, would be to quickly find and get a director's position. In the mornings, I told myself I had to keep busy and give full attention to my daily work at the office, just to take my mind off that devastating feeling of disappointment. Finally, one of my colleagues, who had just accepted a director's position in a distant city, told me of another position in exurbia, where he had been recently interviewed, but without success. I called up and was asked to submit a resume, and within the next two weeks, I had an interview with an Assistant Administrator and with the Medical Director of that hospital. During a brief tour of the Department of Pathology and Laboratory, I noticed that the director was still there, but I was not introduced to him. I had a feeling that he did not know I was a candidate for his job.

One week after the interview, I received a letter from the Assistant Administrator, offering me the Director's position, with a salary of 80,000 and a contract. I signed and mailed back the contract as fast as I could. I was on a rebound and began to sleep much better. It was May of 1977, only two months after that awful rejection. The new position fit my professional expectations, though it was in a relatively remote exurban area. However, we would live in a region which hopefully had some decent public schools, clean air, and very affordable real estate. Not too far away were a few excellent colleges and some significant industries, and one could expect that the area might have some cultural events despite being quite far from any large city.

The story with Mr. Adams had a little sequel about nine months later. By then, my mind had healed from the fiasco, and I was completely enveloped in my new job as Director of Pathology and Laboratory. One morning at work, my secretary gave me a long-distance call from Philadelphia. I picked up the phone, wondering who could that be? There was a female voice:

"Hello, Dr. Yellinek! This is Ruth Werner. I am the pathologist from Philadelphia. We spoke once, about a year ago, when you were applying for a position with Mr. Adams, the administrator…"

"Yes! I remember very well! Hello! How are you?"

"You know, I still have friends at that hospital, and I heard from Dr. Smith what happened to you. He sent me a copy of your resume. I now need a partner at work, and I thought of you. You would work as a co-director with me. It's a nice hospital in a suburb of Philadelphia, and the salary—" but I did not want her to go on, and interrupted:

"Sorry! I thank you, but I am all settled! I appreciate very much that you thought of me, and really, I thank you for the offer! Since we are talking, I would still like to know, what was the reason that you left that hospital?"

"Well, now I don't mind telling you. Both of us, pathologists found that Adams was receiving kickbacks on purchases of lab equipment. We knew too much, and Adams got a wind of it, and we both were dismissed!"

"Well, I am learning! Thanks again for your offer, and good luck with your search!"

"Thank you! Goodbye now. Maybe our paths will cross again." It was nice to hear that, but we never met again.

There was yet another epilogue to this story. About six months later, at the annual meeting and lectures of the College of American Pathologists in San Francisco, in a large meeting hall I saw a young pathologist wearing a badge of the hospital where I met Mr. Adams. I approached the pathologist, introduced myself, and said:

"So, how are things going at your hospital?"

"Well, how do you know of our hospital?"

"A while ago, I meant to take a job there!"

"Well, for now, things are OK! Recently though, our director suffered a severe heart attack, and he will not come back to work. We now have a temporary locum tenens pathologist, who, we hope, might stay on as our director. And we also have a new administrator."

"Really? And where is Mr. Adams?"

"You know him? He resigned."

"Well, nice to have met you! Enjoy the lectures!" It was nice to know that Adams was no longer there.

The other job interview which I will never forget, happened more than ten years later, in 1988, when I was trying to get a director's position closer to a large urban center. It gave me yet another experience that will forever vividly reside in my memory. It began when I answered an ad for a director's position in a downtown Philadelphia hospital and got invited for an interview with the Medical Board. The interview went well, and I was given a tour of the laboratory and pathology facilities. My checking into the hospital's financial stability was satisfactory; the hospital registry showed that it had very few empty beds, and the records showed that the patient census throughout several past years was stable. The building was rather old, but appeared well- maintained, and it was partially renovated. The equipment in the lab and in the X-ray department was modern and new. I felt that the hospital, despite being in a large city with lots of competition, was 'viable'. The Chairman of the Medical Board informed me that there was "a fair number of candidates" to be interviewed and that it might take a while before a decision would be forthcoming. More than six weeks passed by, and I began to expect the usual letter to let me know that the position had been filled.

Another three weeks passed, and unexpectedly, I received a letter from the Chairman of the Medical Board, informing me that I should call him to schedule a second interview, this time, with the hospital's Governing Board. I understood that I was seriously considered for the job; the Governing Board is usually composed of well-heeled, respectable businessmen, usually including some hospital benefactors and the Chairman of the Medical Board.

The interview was set at a downtown business office of one of the Board members. I took a day off, drove into Philadelphia and stayed overnight to be fresh for the interview in the morning. At the given downtown address, the doorman directed me to the anteroom of the Board meeting. Arriving there, a secretary offered me coffee while I waited to be called into the Board room. Soon, I was ushered into a large room where about twelve people sat around a long conference table. I was offered a seat at one end of that table, facing the Chairman of the Governing Board, who was seated far at the opposite end. The Chairman of the Medical Board, the only person I knew from the first interview, introduced me, and the members of the Governing Board introduced themselves. Going around the table, each member started asking questions, mainly probing my management skills.

They were apparently all businessmen and were not very interested in my professional background. This went on for about 45 minutes and then there was a break, and I was asked to wait in the anteroom and have some coffee and cake.

It did not take long, and I was called back into the conference room. I sat in my place at one end of the long table, and the Chairman of the Governing Board said that they decided to offer me the director's position, but, before discussing the remuneration and the benefits package, they wanted me to learn a little more about the background and history of the hospital. He continued with a detailed presentation, revealing that the hospital was an old, established and respectable downtown institution with a very long tradition. That was followed by more information about the sound financial position and the future building and development plans which were approved by the city council, and other positive developments… Suddenly, I heard a word that struck me like lightning! The Chairman was saying that the relations between the hospital management and the union were very good. Upon hearing the word "union", I could feel the blood surging into my face, and I leaned back into my seat. One of the Board members, sitting close to me, looked straight at my face and quietly said:

"You are changing colors! Are you alright?" There was a little pause. I had to collect myself before answering:

"Yes… I am OK!" – and I swallowed, but my mouth was completely dry. The Chairman, meanwhile, had stopped talking, and I realized that even from the far end of the table, he must have seen the red glow on my face.

"Do you need a little water?" he asked.

"No, thank you!" I finally composed myself:

"It is just that…, you mentioned the union…, and my experience with the union +was not so good!" I paused, and then explained:

"Just hearing the word 'union' reminds me of it! It's a reflex."

"Do you mind telling us what happened?" the Chairman asked.

"No! Of course, I can tell you." My mouth was still dry, and I asked:

"May I, please, have a cup of water?"

The secretary was called, and she brought me a cup of water. I took a few sips and felt the blood slowly draining down from my face. I knew that my color was returning to normal, and I was well. I had to think fast: *This job, though very desirable only a few minutes ago, now seemed much less so… I had to make an instant decision! Do I want to work with a union? In a flash, I decided I no longer wanted that position.*

I took my time to tell them the whole story, how, in a previous position in NYC, a union member sued me for "discrimination by color", and although the lawsuit was dismissed, I decided to stay away from any hospital, that allowed a union to have an influence on the function of the medical personnel. I explained that in my current position I worked for a hospital that has been actively keeping the union out! In the end, I just said:

"I am sorry, but I cannot accept the position you are offering. I thank you very much for your time!"

While I was talking, the Chairman of the Board kept nodding, and then he went:

"I understand you, but please, tell us, why do you feel so strongly about the union?"

"Well, it has to do with the attitude of a union worker. It may be alright in an industrial plant, where no one gets hurt if the workers walk out and the production of some widgets is disrupted. But, in a hospital? I have seen union workers in the hospital dropping everything and leaving the minute their shift was over. This is not acceptable in a medical lab, nor is it compatible with a nurse's job, nor with any medical duty."

"Well, we appreciate you being so candid about it." said the Chairman.

"I apologize for taking so much of your time, and I do thank you for your consideration."

"Well, good luck to you!" said the Chairman of the Board.

"Thank you! Goodbye!" and I got up and left.

Today, 35 years later, new circumstances have driven even the physicians to join the union, and with good reason!

As I walked out into the cool city air, the bitter taste of the union completely cleared out of my mind. I felt a relief and even satisfaction from having rejected that job. I walked through the city, looked at some shop windows, and suddenly felt hungry; it was lunchtime. I was in Philly many times before, attending ECOG and other pathology meetings, and I knew of some decent restaurants. I started walking towards one of them, and the thought about the end of the interview returned to me with a certain pleasure. Yes, it was a good decision! Anyway, a job in the middle of a large, crowded city was perhaps not the best choice, but working with a union around my neck was surely not a position I would want to take. There would be other, better opportunities coming up, and I needed only one...

After lunch, I had a long drive home, and while driving, I thought of the very recent unsolicited job offer that I had only two months earlier and declined to accept. That offer came from my old research mentor, Yoshi Komura, who in the meantime had become a tenured Professor and Chairman of the Department of Pathology at a medical school in Southern California. He was looking for a Director of Pathology and Laboratory in a newly built hospital, affiliated with his medical school. Yoshi had tracked me down and reached me by phone, and I agreed to check out his offer. He sent me an airline ticket with a hotel reservation for a three-day visit, giving me a chance to assess the job and the conditions in the beautiful Orange County. I flew into John Wayne Airport, stayed in a posh hotel, and saw the newly built hospital and its administrator. The hospital was almost finished, and the position offered a very good remuneration. The clinical lab and the pathology department, though amply proportioned and well equipped, were placed deep below ground, next to the morgue, and without a single window.

That location was depressing, and it was the first thing that turned me off. The lavish hotel also did not impress me favorably. All people working in the lobby were fair skinned, including the tall, blond girls doing shoe-shine service and serving food in the cafeteria and the restaurant. Peeking behind the cafeteria kitchen door, I saw only people of color, working the jobs behind the scenes. Walking through the streets of a privately owned town, I saw notices announcing unusual restrictions. It was explained to me that in a privately owned town, the owners had the right to make all the rules. On the last evening, at dinner with Yoshi and his wife in a fine Japanese restaurant, he told me that despite his high position at the medical school, he had to put up a fight to be allowed to join the local golf club. The club management had to make for him "an exception". As soon as I returned home, I called Yoshi and thanked him for the offer and for his hospitality. I did not think we would fit into that part of California. All throughout Orange County I felt the spirit of the John Birch Society, which made me think of another, much earlier experience in California.

It was back in the late seventies when, after attending a professional meeting in San Francisco, I took a few days of vacation to see and explore the coast of California. I rented a car and drove all the way down to San Diego and even further, into Mexico. Driving along the scenic coastal road and listening to the radio constantly repeating the same popular song, "It Never Rains in Southern California", I decided to stay overnight in Santa Barbara. Once there, in every motel with a lit-up "vacancy" sign, as soon as I walked in, the clerk quickly turned off the vacancy sign and said something like:

"Esta lleno!" or "Sorry, we are full!"

Most motel clerks greeted me and spoke to me in Spanish. I understood: a person with black, curly hair, short stature, wearing old blue jeans and an open shirt was expected to speak only Spanish and would not be trusted with a motel room. After four such failures to get a room, I entered the next motel and introduced myself very loudly, practically yelling:

"Dr. Yellinek from New York!", and like a miracle, the desk clerk spoke English and promptly put a room key on the counter. A doctor from New York was acceptable, and his outward appearance did not matter. Santa Barbara appeared to be a charming town, but the atmosphere in it felt stale. It was a town, where it's nice to make a day visit, but I would not want to live there.

On that same trip, I spent a day in Mexico and stayed overnight in a motel on the beach in Ensenada. Just wanted to check, if the Pacific there was any warmer than in San Francisco. Not much, perhaps by one degree. After about five minutes of swimming, my skin felt as if it had been rubbed with sandpaper, and I had to quickly get out of the water and dry myself. Later in the evening, while dining in a restaurant, next to my table sat an American family with three children aged between about 8 and 12. When I overheard one of the children saying something cute, I gave a little laugh, and the father of the family noticed. He looked at me with expression of surprise and said:

"You understand English?"

"Why not?"

"Sorry! I thought you were from here."

"I am from New York!" - and then we chatted a little across the table.

That nice family was from Southern California, and of course, to them, I looked like a person who should speak Spanish. So, I came to understand that in California I was supposed to be Hispanic. I already knew that on the East Coast, many people took me simply for a 'person of color'.

The drive home from Philadelphia dragged on, and my memory turned a little further back into the mid-seventies, around 1976, the time when I was about to leave my academic career and seek my first position as Director of Pathology. At that time too, I had an unsolicited job offer which I declined. A colleague from my residency training days, Albert Kaplan called me one evening and offered a full partnership position in his pathology corporation in Little Rock, AK. The position had a very lucrative revenue arrangement that would immediately more than triple my income. We spoke on the phone for over an hour, but I could only say to Albert that I did not think Miriam would want to move so far away from NYC. Despite my reluctance, a few days later, the postman brought a thick certified letter containing airline tickets for Miriam and me, with a letter, inviting us to visit over the coming four-day Memorial Day weekend and stay in Albert's home without any obligation to accept the job, and, as Albert wrote, "just to have a good time together". Miriam and I needed no more than five minutes to decide that it would not be right to accept Albert's offer, and I mailed back the airline tickets. I also immediately called Albert on the phone, thanked him, and explained that we already had plans for that Memorial Day weekend and that anyway, we preferred to live closer to the East Coast.

The real reason for our decision was the well-known 1954 school incident in Little Rock, AK, which required President Eisenhower's intervention. That event was firmly imprinted in our memories, and both of us felt a real concern over how our family would be treated in Arkansas. Now I know that we made the right decision, because even today, more than 50 years later, the conditions have remained such that we still wouldn't want to live in any part of the South or certain parts of the Mid-West. We never visited Albert but continued to stay in touch over the next several years. Four years later, Albert's wife sadly let us know that he had succumbed to a malignant melanoma (cancer of skin).

* * *

I came home from Philadelphia late in the evening, tired from a long drive, and it was a pleasure to be welcomed by Miriam. She did not mind that I returned empty-handed and would have to continue the search for a new position.

That search ended the following year, in 1989, shortly after I had a very plain and easy interview with two young administrators of a large suburban hospital. It was the very last time that I interviewed for a job. Despite the dark predictions from my good friends, and despite my 'advanced age', I received the position of Director of the Department of Pathology and Laboratory for the second time in my career. That position would last for well over a dozen years and it would be more challenging than any of my previous engagements.

Chapter 14

Hospital Administrators

In my travel through several hospital positions, I met several administrators, and each one was different. My first encounter with a hospital administrator was when I became an intern in NYC and tried to rent a small studio apartment near the hospital. A relatively large cash deposit of 200 dollars was required up-front, and only two and a half months after our arrival into US, it was well beyond our means. The apartment was very conveniently located, and it was "rent-controlled", meaning that the monthly rent was quite low (80 dollars). Such apartments were hard to find, and I was desperately trying to quickly make a deposit before someone else did. I went to the office of the hospital administrator, Mr. Constantine, a tall, middle-aged man with greying hair and a rather kind face. In my heavily accented, broken English, I asked him if it were possible to get a loan from the hospital. A whole head taller than I, he looked at me from above and started shaking his head and smiling. He must have been amused, both with the unusual request and with my accent. Then he said:

"A loan? But we are not a bank!"

I looked at him, not knowing what to say. At that moment, his face, with a long, pointy nose and cunning grey eyes reminded me of a weasel, and though I did not feel like smiling, I gave him a forced smile. There was an awkward pause, after which he said:

"OK! Come with me!"

He walked out into the hallway, and I followed. He went down the hall to a little glass window, where a lady greeted us with:

"Hello! How may I help?"

"Hi! We need two hundred! Cash, please!" said Mr. Constantine, and then, turning to me, he explained:

"The cashier will give you the money, and now you'll have to work very hard! Over the next eight months, twenty-five dollars will be deducted from your salary!"

"Thank you very much!"

"OK! We are glad to help!" And he rushed back to this office.

I was standing by the cashier's window, overwhelmed by a feeling of gratefulness and happiness. It was only my third month in America, and to see such kindness was a pleasure! The lady behind the glass window copied my name off the badge on my coat and, through a slit under the glass, pushed toward me two bills of one hundred dollars. Two such large bills I had never seen or held in my hand! My bi-weekly salary check was about 120 dollars. Well, it was 1962, and a first-class postage stamp cost five cents.

Fifteen years later, Mr. Loughlin, the administrator who hired me into my first position as Director of Pathology, reminded me of Mr. Constantine. During the one year I worked under him, he never said a false word, he gave straight answers, and he made decisions which were as close to 'fair' as possible. I was taught from early on in my life that there was no such thing as 'fairness', especially not in business.

In my second year at that hospital, Mr. Loughlin, unfortunately, left for another position. Another young man, Mr. Panartios, was hired and put in charge of the laboratory and pathology. Mr. Panartios, a tall, lean man in his late thirties, appeared pleasant and personable, and as we sometimes sat for lunch at the same table in the cafeteria, he confided some of his personal issues. He brought to town his wife with two children and an elderly widowed father, who was very ill. His father used to be a heavy smoker, and about two years earlier, he was diagnosed with cancer of the lung. The way his cancer was discovered, and what followed, was an interesting story.

One evening, at dinner in a restaurant, Mr. Panartios's father started choking. A chicken bone was stuck in his throat, and he was urgently taken to a nearby doctor's office. An ENT specialist took an X-ray and quickly extracted the chicken bone. About a year later, his father started having a severe cough which lasted over a month, and when a chest X-ray was taken in a Baltimore hospital, it revealed a tumor in the lung. It turned out to be cancer. My friendly administrator demanded a review of the X-ray taken in the ENT specialist's office, and it was found that along with the chicken bone in the esophagus, there was also a small, very faint shadow in the lung, which at the time was not noticed. The ENT specialist was sued for malpractice, and Mr. Panartios won a large reward for his father. I felt sorry for the clinician who in an emergency missed seeing a barely visible tiny shadow in the lung. I did not like the whole story.

Within several months, Mr. Panartios's father was admitted to our hospital, and within two weeks, he passed away. I was asked to do an autopsy, and after a very long and thorough examination, I could not find any residual cancer in multiple sections, not even a microscopic trace. In place of the lung tumor, there was a solid mass of dense scar tissue, and I also found pervasive scaring throughout the entire remaining lung. Apparently, all cancer tissue had been destroyed by a combination of chemotherapy and radiation. Upon having read my full autopsy report, Mr. Panartios wanted to sue the Baltimore oncologists for having destroyed his father's lungs by wrongful therapy. I spent quite some time talking to him to convince him that such autopsy findings were common in patients with lung cancer when they were treated by combined chemotherapy and radiation. It was the only treatment available at that time, and it prolonged his father's life for at least two years; without it, he would have died much sooner.

Despite our apparent friendship and confidence, when the time came for my annual review and salary adjustment, Mr. Panartios awarded me a two percent increase. I asked for a formal appointment to speak to him about it, and he received me very cordially:

"Hi Peter, what can I do for you?"

"Well, I'd like to talk about my annual review. How do you feel about my performance? Did you find any problem?"

"Oh, no! You have been doing very well, and Mr. Loughlin also left very favorable notes about your work."

"Well, as you know, this year, the inflation has reached into double digits. My annual raise is two percent. That puts the value of my salary way below that of last year."

Mr. Panartios looked at me for a few seconds with a strange expression. Then he began to speak, loudly annunciating every word:

"Well, you know, as a physician, you are already earning a very high salary! You really do not need more money!" and he emphasized the word "more".

I was stunned by his attitude. I could only say:

"Well, if you feel that way…, thanks for your time!"

I began to realize what kind of person this administrator really was. Behind his facade of friendship, he harbored some unsavory personal beliefs. He was one of those people who carried a feeling that the physicians, and all professionals except managers were overpaid. At that moment, I chose not to make any further issue of it. I decided to wait for an opportunity to bring it up with the head administrator of the hospital.

A few months later, the wife of Mr. Panartios was hospitalized with pneumonia. During her hospital stay, she was found to have a fungus infection in one eye, and by the time she was discharged from the hospital, she had a severe loss of vision in that eye. Notwithstanding his position at the hospital, Mr. Panartios sued both the hospital and every one of the physicians who participated in the care of his wife. He and his lawyer accused the hospital and the physicians of negligent treatment, causing the infection and severe loss of her vision.

The administrator was summarily fired, and the case was settled out of court for an undisclosed sum. Before leaving the hospital, Mr. Panartios had the gall to come to me, ostensibly to say goodbye, and then he asked whether I knew of any job opening for a hospital administrator. I told him to check the newspapers. Three months later, I heard that he was again employed as an administrator at a hospital in New England. There must have been a terrible shortage of hospital managers.

A young nun, a trainee/administrator who I met in my first job as a director of the department, had a real talent for her profession, and she certainly acted as a smart, tough manager. She taught me that a manager must think with his head and not with his heart, and ten years later, she became the head administrator of a large hospital. The senior nun and head administrator who handled my crisis with the Medical Director, Dr. Blusher, proved to be both wise and consistent and steady in her role of a hospital administrator.

In my overall experience with hospital administrators, I was quite lucky. Both Mr. Constantine and Mr. Loughlin were not only easy to work with, but they were both smart and decent people. On the other hand, Panartios was an example of a nasty manager, somewhat like Mr. Adams, who caused me only aggravation. The other few administrators that I dealt with through all those years were capable managers: crafty, smart, sometimes rough and at other times polished, always behaving as needed, and habitually evasive and blank-faced.

Chapter 15

"The Second Time is Easy"

In January of 1990, following a week of vacation on a Caribbean island, I started a new position as Director and Chairman of the Department of Pathology and Laboratories at a hospital located in quiet suburban backwoods, about 70 minutes away from a major city. The old retiring director had been in that position for over twenty years, and when I took over, it was evident that for the past ten years he had been coasting along without any care to keep up with the time.

I found everything in manual mode. The pathology office used typewriters with blue carbon copy paper to issue pathology reports. Not even word processors were used. Numerous large drawers contained paper files with copies of old reports from the last five years; older files were available in a basement storage room. Microscopic slides were made in a sloppy manner, allowing the possibility of cross-contamination by tissue particles, a most dangerous practice. The clinical lab was run by a manager who leased a chemistry analyzer that was notorious for its unstable test results, thus requiring constant labor-intensive adjustments.

The department had two assistant pathologists who had been there for several years, and one of them, Dr. Pangalan, had applied for the director's position but failed to get it. The latter one met me, oozing artifice of sweetness and repeatedly expressing his "great relief" over my arrival. The other assistant pathologist, Dr. Pumaren, appeared reticent, and he eventually turned out as a trustworthy associate. Though both were immigrants from the same country, I soon found out that my two assistant pathologists were, for some reason not on good speaking terms, and it was not because each came from a different clan and spoke a different dialect. It appeared that the two were simply made of a different fabric.

Not long before I started this job, I was told that after twelve and a half years of experience as a director of pathology, doing the same job for a second time should be easy. But the job was in a different environment, with a different staff, and in a large, crowded suburban area. From the very first week I had to tackle one new, unexpected problem after another, and at least some were instigated by the assistant pathologist, who failed in his bid to become director of the department.

The first glaring problem that I immediately recognized was in cytology. The lab had one experienced cytology screener, Tony Torchia, who took care of all fluid cytology and PAP smears. I was informed that he was "a true professional" with an excellent reputation and "impeccable diagnostic skills". He had over 25 years of experience, and his knowledge of cytology was described as "better than that of a pathologist".

I soon found out, what the source of Tony's high proficiency was. Every morning, he arrived at work very early, at 6:30 am, and he would first collect the list of patients whose fluid cytology he was to screen that day. Then, he would go on the hospital floors and read the X-ray reports and all other clinical records of those patients. So informed and biased by the clinical information, he would be able to screen the microscopic slides very quickly and promptly telephone his findings to the clinicians. A pathologist would later review Tony's preliminary screening assessment and issue a proper, signed diagnostic report. My predecessor, Dr. Farber, allowed this practice and comfortably enjoyed Tony's prowess.

Within the first few days on the job, I told Tony that no information should be passed on to a clinician before one of the pathologists reviewed the microscopic slides and signed the official report. Tony did not seem happy about it, but nevertheless, said he would comply. However, he quickly informed the clinicians about the new policy, and the clinicians got upset and complained to the hospital administration that my new policy would cause a delay in treatment of their patients. Very soon, I was called to a meeting with the hospital administrator to explain the issue. He grasped the legal liability of Tony's practice and suggested that I set up a special meeting with clinicians of all specialties that used cytology services.

Prior to setting up that meeting, I asked one of the thoracic surgeons whether he felt that it was proper to get a diagnostic report from a screener, a technologist, and act upon it before a review by a pathologist, a licensed physician. He looked at me with an expression as if I was out of my mind. He then exclaimed:

"Are you kidding me? And what's wrong with that? This guy, Tony, knows more cytology than a pathologist! Why should I have my treatment delayed just so that one of your assistants may sign the report? Anyway, Tony is so experienced that the final reports always confirm his diagnosis."

"Well, this may be true in most cases, but what would happen if the pathologist's diagnosis was different? Both you and the hospital would have the liability of a malpractice case!" I failed to add that I, as director of the department, would also be liable.

"But such a thing has never happened!" he retorted.

"The hospital administration will soon call a meeting to go over this issue." It was clear that I was disturbing a normal, well-established routine; I dared to 'upset the apple cart'.

The meeting with the surgeons, gynecologists, internists, pulmonary specialists and some other clinicians was set up for an early morning, at 7 am, so as not to interfere with their busy surgical schedule. From the outset, the meeting did not go well. I started by presenting two simple points:

1. Technologists are not licensed to practice medicine, and they should not provide a report to a clinician before a pathologist reviews and signs it.
2. A clinician acting upon a report from a technologist might be exposed to the liability of malpractice.

Several clinicians, obviously tipped off by Tony, started immediately showering me with contrary comments and questions:

"Tony is an expert cytologist; he's always been right with his diagnosis!"

"Always?" I asked.

"Why are you so set against Tony?"

"Dr. Farber, the previous director, fully trusted him!"

"Perhaps, but such practice is not legal!"

"We need the diagnosis promptly in the morning, before surgery!"

"We have to keep our schedule!" chimed in another one.

"We cannot have our cytology reports delayed!" clamored a third one.

"Listen, please! I will have the cytologic diagnosis called directly to you, to each one of you, and as early as possible in the morning, I promise!" Some of the physicians started noisily talking among themselves, and I soon felt that it was best to adjourn the meeting and let them go start their busy day.

As I was leaving the meeting, walking next to me was a senior internist, the chief of pulmonary service, and he started talking to me:

"You know, Tony really does get his diagnosis right on the spot, although… well…, we do have here in town… a couple of patients, who are still moving around…", and he stopped walking, and looked at me. Then he continued walking and quietly said, as if speaking to himself:

"…permanently cured." and he followed it with a little snort of suppressed laughter. I understood perfectly well, what he meant, and answered:

"Well, that doesn't surprise me! Tony may be clever and experienced, but he is not a trained pathologist!"

After the meeting, I realized that at no time did any one clinician indicate that he agreed with or accepted my new policy. But at least they were put on notice about the need for a proper, legal way of reporting cytology. Tony's reports were "usually right", but it was clear from the pulmonary specialist's comment that on a few occasions, he provided a "Mickey Mouse" report.

Tony had ingrained habits, and he was very close to retirement, and so, several months later, I was happy to receive his resignation. I hired a new, experienced cytologist, one who followed the rules of proper practice. In the end, the cytology service functioned in a legal manner and without causing any major delay in patient therapy.

A new director of pathology will always have the hardest time during the first three months on the job, when everyone tries to check him out, to see whether he measures up to the task. Along with the controversy about the cytology service, I soon became aware that one of my assistant pathologists, Dr. Pangalan, was casting rumors and innuendos about my work.

This became evident from little remarks and questions coming from a few members of the medical staff, and it came to a culmination when a brash young surgeon, Dr. Brennan one morning met me in the doctors' lounge and challenged my diagnosis of breast cancer in one of his patients. He let me know that Dr. Pangalan thought that his patient who I diagnosed with cancer - had only a benign tumor. He asked me to review the microscopic slides one more time and let him know the outcome. I said I would.

Back in my office, after I calmed down, I called Dr. Pangalan and asked him to review the microscopic slides of that patient together with me on the double-headed microscope. Pointing to a specific area on one of the slides, I asked:

"What do you think of this, here?"

"Yeah, there might be a few atypical cells, but I don't think it's malignant, because most of it, all around, is a benign tumor, a fibroadenoma."

I moved the microscopic slide to another area, near the very edge of the tissue, and asked:

"And what about this area, right here?"

"Yeah, well…, this seems like a little spot of cancer."

"It seems? Or is it cancer?"

"Yeah, well, it is a little area of cancer."

"Shouldn't we tell this to Dr. Brennan?" And I picked up the phone, called Dr. Brennan, and told him that Dr. Pangalan would like to speak to him. Then, while passing the receiver to Dr. Pangalan, I said:

"Now, please, tell Dr. Brennan what the diagnosis is on Mrs. X."

Dr. Pangalan, with a shaky voice, relayed to the surgeon that there was cancer, along with a fibroadenoma. Then I asked for the receiver and confirmed with Dr. Brennan that the question of the diagnosis was cleared up. His patient had cancer, and there was also a benign tumor, a fibroadenoma Dr. Pangalan, still standing next to me, said plaintively:

"I am sorry about this misunderstanding! I did not see the little areas on the edge of this one slide; all other slides show only benign fibroadenoma."

"That's why you prepare multiple cuts from the tumors, to have a better chance of finding what's important. In this case, the invasive cancer is the diagnosis that counts. The presence of a benign tumor, a fibroadenoma, and all other benign changes, the cysts and fibrosis in her breast are of no importance."

However, that did not end the case, because rumors go around fast. The rumor of a "false cancer diagnosis" had reached the chief of surgery, Dr. Zengaro, and he wanted to verify the diagnosis by himself. He came the same afternoon into my office and demanded that I send the microscopic slides of that patient for a consultation at Cancer Memorial Hospital in NYC. I was happy to comply. The letter of consultation arrived in about ten days, and it stated that the diagnosis was invasive cancer in a fibroadenoma. I called Dr. Zengaro to come by my office, and I showed him the consultation report.

Having read the diagnosis, he exclaimed:

"In all my years, I have never seen a cancer arising in a benign fibroadenoma! This must be extremely rare!"

"It's not as rare as you may think! Sooner or later, you run into it."

"Well, this is my first…"

"Let me show you something", and I turned around and picked up a journal from the shelf behind me. Just a month earlier, the "Cancer" journal published an article describing a series of more than one hundred and thirty cases of cancer of breast arising in a fibroadenoma. I opened the journal on the first page of the article and showed it to Dr. Zengaro:

"Would you like to take the journal with you and read the article at home?"

"No, thanks!" He glanced at the first page of the article and said:

"I can see it from the title. Still, it's very unusual." He put the journal back on my desk and turned around to leave.

"Yes, it is not very common!"

Within the next two months, I had another very rare case, that time directly with Dr. Zengaro. He had a patient who was referred to his office with a large, fist-size tumor on the back, right next to the left scapula (shoulder blade). The tumor was very hard, and it was firmly attached to all surrounding tissues, so the patient was referred from an internist's office with a diagnosis of probable sarcoma (cancer of connective tissue). Dr. Zengaro operated and sent me a sample biopsy of the tumor for rapid frozen section diagnosis.

It was a harmless benign tumor, with the appearance of a typical elastofibroma. This was a very uncommon tumor that I had seen in all my years in practice only about five or six times, the first of which was during my training at Columbia University. I reported the diagnosis over the intercom to Dr. Zengaro in the operating room, and he asked:

"What's that? 'Elasto'… what? Say that again!"

"Elastofibroma. It is a benign tumor of connective tissue, composed of a massive overgrowth of elastic fibers."

"You're sure, it's benign? It's hard like a rock and it is firmly invasive into all neighboring tissues, feels like a typical cancer! It must be a malignancy! Are you sure, I don't have to do a radical excision with a wide margin?"

"I am sure, it's benign! It's enough if you take out just the tumor. You don't need a wide margin!"

"Well…, if you say so…" he sounded doubtful.

"These tumors are extremely rare in the US; they are commonly found in Japan, and mostly in women!"

"Thank you."

After surgery, Dr. Zengaro came to my office and asked to see the frozen section of the tumor under the microscope. While he was looking at it, he quietly commented:

"It's another first for me! How do you manage to find these pink elephants?"

"I guess, it's just a lucky thing - especially for the patient!"

"By the way, the patient is Japanese…, and a woman!"

"Well, then it's not at all so unusual! Tomorrow, I will have the slides treated with a special stain for elastic fibers, and you may come and see. The whole tumor will be highly positive." But the busy surgeon never came to see the special stain.

About the same time, though, I had another unpleasant, nasty issue hanging over my head. Dr. Mandel, a middle-aged attending physician and chief of rehabilitation service, had a lump in the thyroid gland removed by a senior surgeon, Dr. Drumarsky. A tumor, or any tissue from a physician is customarily attended to by the director of pathology, and I had the misfortune of having to issue the diagnosis of cancer of thyroid. Understandably, Dr. Mandel was not happy with such a diagnosis, and he immediately had some doubt about it, because cancer of thyroid is known to occur only very rarely in a male. He rightfully requested copies of microscopic slides and took them for a second opinion consultation at a nearby medical school.

The next day, a senior pathologist, professor at the medical school issued a diagnosis of "adenoma of thyroid", a benign tumor. The surgeon, Dr. Drumarsky and I were promptly informed about the discrepancy in diagnosis. I then told both Dr. Mandel and Dr. Drumarsky that additional copies of microscopic slides would be immediately mailed for a consultation with two nationally renowned experts for tumors of the thyroid gland. Of course, when a discrepancy, such as a "false cancer diagnosis", happens to a hospital staff physician, the rumors, questioning the competence of the pathologist will immediately begin to circulate through the entire hospital staff...

One set of microscopic slides I sent to an expert at the University of Pennsylvania, who had written a book and published multiple articles about thyroid tumors, and the other set of slides I mailed to an expert at Harvard Medical School, who also wrote a book on thyroid tumors and published many articles on the subject. Then I waited... Every expert consultant, often a professor of pathology at a medical school, is usually very busy, and consequently, more than two long weeks passed before both consultation letters came back, one following a day after the other. Meanwhile, the ugly, disparaging rumors kept percolating all around me.

Both consultants independently made a diagnosis of cancer of the thyroid gland. I first called the patient, my colleague Dr. Mandel, and gave him all the documentation, and the same day, his wife drove him to Cancer Memorial Hospital in NYC, to begin therapy. The surgeon, Dr. Drumarsky, was also provided with copies of the consultants' reports. Very slowly, the final facts about this case permeated through the members of the medical staff, and I could sense around me a palpably improved attitude, and even a bit of respect.

Gradually, I began to see signs of being accepted by the members of the medical staff. A few of the members, those who were inclined to be more friendly, let me know that they felt bad about an earlier "misunderstanding".

Soon came another case that would also end up reverberating around the hospital staff, this time again initiated by my assistant, Dr. Pangalan. It began on a quiet morning when the chief of family practice, Dr. Bergson visited my office. He walked in and asked me to review a couple of microscopic slides that represented cytologic smears from one of his patients. He stated that the smears were obtained by needle aspiration of a tumor of breast in a middle-aged woman. I examined the two slides, which were obviously made in our lab, and told him that the tumor was benign, most likely caused by a combination of sclerosing adenosis with a cyst and some fat necrosis, or any similar degenerative process. Dr. Bergson looked at me with an expression of doubt:

"Are you sure? Nothing else?"

"Absolutely! I don't see anything worrisome", I replied, "but if you have some doubt, I can send the two slides for a consultation at the Cancer Memorial Hospital. Let me take a moment to check the copy of our report!"

"I have the report right here!" and he handed me a folded sheet of paper. I opened it and saw the diagnosis: ***"Positive for malignant*** *cells"*, signed by Dr. Pangalan. Dr. Bergson looked at me and asked me to close the door of my office. As soon as I shut the door, he said:

"Well, let me sit down and tell you…" He sat on a chair and went on: "The smears… actually…, they belong to my wife! She is the patient!" he paused, and then continued:

"She recently felt a lump in her breast, and I, too, could feel it. We went to Dr. Brennan, and he did a needle aspiration of it, and made two smears and sent them to your lab for cytology."

"Please excuse me, just a few more moments!" I turned around to have another look through the microscope. Dr. Bergson continued:

"The report from your lab says, 'positive for malignant cells', and you are now saying, it's benign?"

"Yes, but please, give me a few more minutes. I want to review the smears one more time."

"Just to let you know, Dr. Brennan has already reserved the time in the operating room. Tomorrow morning, he wants to do a biopsy and send it for a frozen section, and then a mastectomy." (=removal of the breast)

I finished reviewing the slides for a second time, and there was absolutely nothing malignant in them. So, I said:

"Dr. Bergson! Just to assure you, I will now dictate a corrected report with a benign diagnosis, and I will sign it. You will have it in a few minutes, and then you may go home and relax. I will also mail these two slides for a consultation at Cancer Memorial Hospital."

For a few more moments, Dr. Bergson sat quietly in his chair. Then he got up and asked if he could use my office phone. He called Dr. Brennan's office, got his secretary, and left a message for Dr. Brennan to postpone the scheduled surgery on his wife because he wanted to have a consultation with another pathologist. Then he let out a long sigh, and I could see that he was relieved.

When Dr. Bergson left, I took the two microscopic slides, stepped into Dr. Pangalan's office, and asked him to review the case with me on the double-headed microscope. He immediately remembered the patient and told me that Tony had screened the slides and reported malignant cells. He then explained:

"I fully trust Tony's diagnosis! You might not even need to look at the slides!"

"You signed out the case as malignant without looking at the slides?"
"No, no! I mean, Tony is so experienced that one wouldn't have to do much checking after him!" he paused and immediately continued:

"Of course, I checked the slides!"

I put one of the two slides under the double-headed microscope and said:

"Let's now look at the slides together, and thoroughly. You move the slide around, and please, show me the malignant cells..."

He slowly moved the slide, stopping at each cell marked by Tony's ink dot, and booth of us looked. The marked cells were quite enlarged and degenerated, and they looked quite abnormal. Not one of those ink-marked cells had the true characteristics of malignancy, though they had enlarged nuclei and did not appear normal. After having passed every marked cell, Dr. Pangalan said:

"These are abnormal but are not the right ones. The malignant cells must be on the other slide! Let's look there."

We looked at the second slide. After a thorough search and survey of all marked cells, we saw more of the same: very degenerated cells, but none were truly malignant. We both lifted our heads from the microscope, and I said:

"You reported malignant cells, and the patient has been scheduled to have cancer surgery. That's not good! We should talk about this later. Let's meet at the end of the day, at 5 pm, in my office."

"These cells are very abnormal. Tony put them down as malignant, and I felt that…"

"Let's meet at 5!"

"I'll wait for you."

I took the two slides to have them packaged and mailed out with the usual letter of request for consultation.

I was shaken up and had to draw on all my experience. What just happened was reminiscent of the event that occurred at my first job as director. The assistant pathologist had to be asked to resign. And I also remembered the advice from a young nun administrator, how one should act with the head… The current incident showed either negligence or incompetence. Dr. Pangalan either did not bother to look at the slides, because he fully trusted Tony's report, or he did look at the slides, and made a grave error, perhaps because he believed more in Tony's experience than to his own eyes. In any case, the outcome was the same: I could no longer allow Dr. Pangalan to practice in my department, and he had to be asked to resign!

I first contacted the hospital administrator and informed him of what transpired, and of the need to have Dr. Pangalan removed from the medical staff. He fully supported my decision. Next, I called the heads of all clinical departments and informed them about the incident and my plan of action. Each of them asked a few questions, and each understood my position, except for the chief of surgery, Dr. Zengaro. He acted as if he were Dr. Pangalan's patron. He asked many probing questions and kept giving me wavering comments about my decision. Finally, he suggested that if Dr. Pangalan had to resign, I should pay him a severance of at least three months of salary. I did not want to quibble about it and agreed. It would only mean that for the following three months I would have to work for two people, but my department would be rid of an assistant who was incompetent and hostile.

At the end of the workday, I met with Dr. Pangalan in my office. I told him that to issue a diagnosis of malignancy when there was no evidence of any cancer cells was a serious error and a completely unacceptable way to practice pathology. I then told him that it would be best for him to resign from the medical staff, effective immediately, and without giving any cause. He seemed totally surprised by my proposition. I added that he would receive three months of severance pay, and then he said:

"Let me think about this ...!"

We both sat, facing each other for a long minute. Suddenly, he stood up and, all excited, shouted:

"NO! WHY should I resign?"

"You signed out a cancer diagnosis, which was false. This is not acceptable from an attending pathologist on the staff of this hospital. As director of this department, I can no longer trust your work! You also know that the patient happens to be the wife of a member of the medical staff. When this mistake becomes known to the rest of the medical staff, who is still going to trust you or this department? It is best that you now resign!"

He kept quiet, and I explained the alternative:

"If you do not resign, you will be dismissed from this department and from the medical staff. All heads of clinical services and the hospital administrator have been advised of this incident, and they support my position. If you get removed from the medical staff, the cause for such action will go onto your record, and it is required that any physician's removal from hospital staff be reported to the State Department of Health, stating the reason. That may have repercussions on your license to practice. That's why it's best that you now submit a letter of resignation, without stating any cause!"

That had an effect, and he said:

"I want to call my wife!"

I asked him to do it right from my office. It was a brief call conducted entirely in the privacy of his native language. When he hung up, he sat down and remained quiet. He said he wanted to think for a few minutes, and then asked for a sheet of paper. He wrote a letter of resignation, effective immediately and without giving a cause. He let me read it and then signed and dated it. I made copies for him and for the medical staff and hospital administration. Amidst all that, I admired his calligraphic handwriting.

In the course of these events, I noticed that the head of thoracic surgery, Dr. Drumarsky, for whatever reason, did not seem to like me. Aside from being one who spread rumors about me, he was regularly lodging complaints against my department, but never by talking to me directly. He repeatedly complained to the hospital administrator that the lab test results arrived in his office too late, or that some test results were altogether missing, or that the blood for transfusion was not available in time for surgery, or that the cytology reports arrived with too much delay, etc... I had to answer and explain to the administrator about every complaint, and I noticed that the administrator was slowly getting tired of it, as if it were all my fault. This had grown into a regular nuisance, and something had to be done about it.

I began to pay attention to the surgical tissue specimens that came to my department from Dr. Drumarsky. I found that he recently removed a whole lobe of lung, apparently for a 'cancer' seen on X-rays. However, the pathologic diagnosis was fungal infection. That patient could have been properly treated without major surgery and without the loss of a quarter of his lung. The correct diagnosis could have been made easily by a needle biopsy of the lesion, and the patient could have been treated with appropriate drugs to suppress the fungal infection. At worst, following proper treatment, only a tiny part of the lung would have been scarred. As required in such instances, I sent the case for review by the standing hospital committee for quality assurance ("Tissue Committee").

Soon thereafter, I noticed another case of Dr. Drumarsky. Again, he removed a lobe of lung, presumably for cancer of the lung. It turned out that the patient already had a cancer of the colon. The lung tumor was clearly a metastasis from the colon, and if the surgeon had checked the patient's clinical history, the unnecessary removal of a lobe of the lung could have been avoided. The patient had an advanced stage of colon cancer, and he would have been better served by palliative treatment, without any surgery. Again, I sent the case for review by the quality assurance committee. Both cases happened within about three months, and I anticipated that Dr. Drumarsky would receive from the Tissue Committee some sharp cautionary letters that would make him stop and think, both about his way of practice and about the lab and pathology services.

The next time I saw Dr. Drumarsky was at the monthly meeting of the medical board of the hospital, which both of us regularly attended. He was standing in a corner of the room, loudly talking to several other board members, and as I approached, it was hard to believe what he was saying. He was praising the laboratory, telling others how much the lab had improved since I became the Director! I was standing by the side and listening with my mouth open. Was it possible that

Drumarsky was making such laudatory statements? This was the same doctor who, only a few months ago, busily spread rumors about the "wrong diagnosis of cancer" made by the Director of Pathology. So it happened that henceforth, if he ever had a problem with the lab, he would call me or come to my office and talk to me directly. This keen thoracic surgeon was made aware that all surgical procedures end up with a piece of tissue, first on the pathologist's cutting desk and then under the microscope.

A few months after these events, one nice morning Dr. Brennan walked into my office and handed me a copy of "Medical Economics", a little monthly, best known as a "throw-away journal". This paper, full of pharmaceutical advertisements, was regularly distributed for free to all staff physicians, and I never bothered to read it. He opened the journal somewhere in the middle, pointed to an article with the title "The Diagnosis", and asked me to read it. There I read, in vivid detail, about a recent incident in some fictitious hospital. The author of the article, though disguised under a pseudonym, had to be Dr. Bergson, and I easily recognized that the whole story was about the incident with his wife. Of course, the location and all physicians' names have been changed. The article also recommended that whenever one receives a diagnosis of cancer, it is best to get a second opinion. I feel that the same advice should be followed by every patient who gets a life-threatening diagnosis of any sort, and, for reasons that need not be elaborated, I would also add: "…and seek that second opinion from a reputable institution located in another, faraway city". That issue of Medical Economics I did not throw away, and I still have it as a souvenir.

After six months in my new position, I was finally free from "fighting fires", and I could begin to make changes in the antiquated pathology department. First, I needed to introduce the much overdue computer age into diagnostic pathology. It was nearly the end of 1990, and I had to convince the administration that using typewriters with blue carbon copy paper (does anyone still remember it?) and stacks of drawers with paper files was thoroughly inefficient and wasteful. It took a whole year to push through that idea and to get the budget approved for a small computer system. The administration allowed a maximum of 20,000 dollars, and I had to do with that. I searched high and low, and toward the end of 1991, I located a small informatics company with a single owner/analyst, who created a bare, rudimentary software for pathology reporting and billing, mounted on antiquated Wang hardware. It was used by only six small pathology departments in and around Chicago. I contacted one of the pathologists, and he, together with the IT owner, agreed to demonstrate the system at his hospital. The list price for the whole system, including software and hardware, was 40,000 dollars, double of my budget, but it was the lowest-priced system I could find. I thought that there was a solution, and with a little invention, it could be done.

In 1992, I spent four days and nights in Oak Park, near Chicago, staying as a guest at the pathologist's home and working at the nearby hospital, where the system was in operation. With my previous background in anatomic pathology software, I showed the owner/analyst how, with a few useful and practical tweaks and additions, the software could be expanded and become much more functional, and thereby of greater value to the user and as well to the owner. While I was there, the analyst quickly built and tested the newly suggested modules, and I let him merge in the CAP database nomenclature, which I owned. The analyst had a much-improved product, and in exchange for my contribution, he agreed to a substantial reduction in the price of his software. Then he located a stash of used Wang computers, which on the market had virtually no value, and the total price came down to within my budget. The analyst loaded the newly designed software into a network of seven Wang machines, and a month later, it all arrived, was installed, tested, and became functional in our pathology office.

To maintain the system, I hired an experienced computer analyst to work part-time on a freelance basis. She had full freedom to choose her work hours, and she performed the system maintenance in the evenings, so there was no downtime during daily work hours. She worked for me for nine years in a most efficient way, and she also ran my private billing. In all those years, the pathology computer was functioning like a clockwork, and it was "down" during the daily work hours only about five or six times, and for no longer than a few minutes.

The introduction of the computer in the pathology office created a problem. The analyst had to train a clerical staff, that never used a computer. It was a daunting task. Despite the utmost patience of the analyst, one of our office clerks just couldn't grasp the essence of computer function. She treated the computer as if it were a typewriter. Each time she made a few errors in the data entry of a patient, she would abandon the messed-up document file and start entering the same patient's data all anew. She acted as if she were discarding a piece of paper from a typewriter and then starting with a new, clean sheet of paper. The result was that the computer database had two or more partial entries for the very same patient, the "orphan" files which hung in the system, and the analyst had to first find them and clean them out.

Finally, I asked the HR department to transfer that office clerk to a different position, and she was placed in the X-ray department. Very soon, the X-ray department was also computerized, and our good office clerk was dismissed. She worked in the pathology office for 26 years and she had a brother who was an attorney. The hospital was served with a lawsuit for "discrimination by age", and it had to settle out of court for a substantial sum. The chief of HR then told the administration that it was all a fault of the director of pathology. Responding to that, I could only suggest, that the problem was created by the choices made in the HR department. This, too, was one of the "little joys" of a director.

When it came to computerizing the large clinical laboratory, the choice of comprehensive software and hardware was made by the hospital's finance department. The upshot was that the hospital received the best possible software for billing, but the laboratory got a mediocre product that lacked the entire blood bank module. Later, when discussing the lab software with the administrator, I had to admit that it was more important for the hospital to have an efficient billing system. The lab would have to make do with whatever it received. It only meant that the blood bank would continue to function by using manual records…

Chapter 16

Lab Inspection and Sundry Tidbits

My State inspection problems began with the advent of a novelty: little test kits designed for instant, "bedside" patient testing. As soon as the doctors learned about these commercially available test kits, they wanted them in the hospital. The kits gave test results that were not as accurate as those done on proper lab equipment, but they were convenient and served for a quick, "ballpark" assessment. In the early nineties, the test kits began to be used by nurses and visiting physicians on all patient floors in the hospital. Within two months, I received notice of a new regulation issued by the State Department of Health, requiring that all patient tests done within hospital premises must have a full set of quality control tests with a permanent record of all results, the same standard as required for tests done by the technologists in the laboratory.*

----

* Hospital laboratories are regularly inspected for compliance with standards of safety and performance mandated by Federal and State authorities. A regular annual inspection is done by an inspector from the State Department of Health. She or he could appear without a warning on any day of the year. The director of laboratory and pathology is responsible that everything is done according to regulations. Since State inspection results are available as a public record, any deficiency may damage the hospital's reputation.

Lab test quality control regulations require that at the beginning of each work shift, every piece of lab equipment must be tested by running each individual test with commercial quality control samples at three different value levels, that is, "high," "normal," and "low." Patient tests may be run only after all three levels of control results show correct values. All control results must be recorded, and all records must be saved and available for inspection.

According to the new regulations, the Director of Laboratory was responsible for the quality controls and records thereof, not only in the laboratory, but also throughout the entire hospital. That added a big burden to my job. How could I enforce the performance of quality control tests by the nurses on all hospital floors? Being in a hurry, the nurses would do the patient tests and record results in the chart, but they often forgot to run the required control tests, or they omitted to record the control results. A lack of that record would be taken by the State inspector, as if no control tests were done at all, and that would be considered as severe deficiency in patient safety.

So it happened that one nice morning in the mid-nineties, the State inspector suddenly walked into the hospital and came straight to my office. He greeted me and told me that he would first check the "bedside testing" on patient floors and would inspect the lab and pathology later. This inspector knew me well from several prior inspections, and on this occasion, prior to the customary final summation conference, he came to my office to discuss his findings on the patient floors. As I feared, he discovered quite a few serious deficiencies, mostly missing records of control tests. The inspection of the lab and pathology was in perfect order. We had a brief discussion about bedside testing, and the inspector decided to "give me a break". He would omit in his report the deficiencies found on hospital floors and in the nursery, since it was a new regulation, and it was also the very first time that those areas were being inspected. His decision was, however, conditional on my promise that the problem would be quickly corrected and would not be allowed to happen again.

At the end of the day, the inspector held the customary summation meeting with all lab supervisors, and as usual, the hospital administrator showed up to hear the results. The inspector presented the findings of his inspection and stated that overall, the lab and pathology passed with an excellent grade. Just before ending the summation, he said, somewhat vaguely, that he did notice certain 'issues' on the hospital floors and in the nursery, but this time, he wouldn't include them in the official report - on account of the new regulations and the pigeons... Ending the summation, he declared that the lab and pathology should be congratulated for their performance. The administrator and all lab supervisors were happy that the inspection passed well, and I was relieved. The administrator seemed to have ignored the inspector's final comment, or rather, he was wise enough not to ask anything about it.

When the inspector departed, the administrator called me into his office and asked:

"Just what did he mean by that... whatever it is, new regulation with pigeons?"

It was a good time to tell him the whole truth: that we had serious deficiencies on the hospital floors and particularly in the nursery, where newborn babies were at risk, and that I needed the administration to enforce proper quality control procedures and full record-keeping by nurses.

"But what does that have to do with pigeons?" the administrator insisted. Then I explained that it was about a story I told the inspector just before the summation conference, and here it is.

NYC had an ordinance that forbids people to feed the pigeons, because they damaged the city buildings. One day, an old lady was sitting on a Central Park bench and throwing food to the birds that were swarming all around her. A policeman appeared and started writing a ticket. The lady protested: 'Officer, I am not feeding the pigeons! I am feeding the sparrows! You try and tell the pigeons to go away!'

I then told the administrator that, obviously, the inspector liked the story, and it made sense: I was not in control of the nurses on hospital floors, and so, this time, the inspector let us off the hook, but for the next time, we better be prepared! The administrator then asked me to give him a few days, and a program for nurses' education would be set in motion and enforced. I thanked him, and within two weeks after the inspection, the nurses were formally educated and began to rigorously maintain all quality control records for bedside testing, as required by State regulations.

* * *

During the 25 years I served as director of a department, I regularly attended the monthly meetings of the hospital Medical Board. Among other issues, I witnessed several bitter turf fights that took place in those meetings. The hospital administration was only interested in having a smooth admission of patients into the hospital, and an administrator would only occasionally have to intervene, to calm the fights between the physicians. Some of those fights were as sharp as if they were between two alpha baboons.

A young general surgeon, who also specialized in urology, joined the medical staff of the hospital, and he immediately received full privileges to admit patients for general surgery. He later applied for privileges in urologic surgery. When his application came for approval at the Department of Urology, the current members of that department managed to find all sorts of excuses to deny him privileges. That group wanted all urologic patients for themselves. It was a clear case of turf protection. This fight between the young surgeon and the old, established urology staff was uneven and unfair, and it lasted for nearly a year.

Amidst those "turf" proceedings, this young surgeon, Dr. Michael Stone, sat one day for lunch at my table in the hospital cafeteria, and in no time, he began to talk about the sore subject, knowing full well that I sat on the Medical Board. As he spoke about his complaint, he got all excited and suddenly came out with the following statement:

"You know, it is very clear to me why they are denying me the privileges in urology! It's all coming from that damn Weaver! He is an antisemite!"

He looked upset and angry, and I thought I'd better be careful and not start laughing. At that moment, he looked like someone who was not ready for any jokes. So, I just calmly said:

"Didn't you know? Dr Weaver is Jewish!"

Hearing this, he was stunned. He looked like just having received a cold shower. Then, with a suspicion in his tone, he asked:

"Are you sure? You wouldn't be kidding me!"

"No, no! You can ask anyone on the staff!"

"Then, why, the hell, does Weaver stand against giving me the privileges in urology?"

"Maybe, because the head of urology is his old friend. Anyway, they claim that you did not have sufficient training in urology. If you can prove that you did, they will have to let you in."

"I gave them my record of training! I am tired of waiting! I'll start suing Weaver and all of them, bastards!"

"I hope it won't go that far!"

Our lunch was over, and we each went our own way. It was funny: Dr. Stone was a very tall guy, blond and blue-eyed, a perfect Nordic type, and with that last name, I had no idea that he was Jewish.

Probably his grandpa's name was Stein. It is well known that many immigrants choose to anglicize their family name; the US allows it right upon entry into the country and as well when issuing the citizenship.

Dr. Stone's adversary, Dr. Jack Weaver, was a general surgeon recruited for this turf fight by the urologists, just to appear as a "neutral" arbitrator. To see if this conflict could come to an end, a few days later, I joined Dr. Weaver for lunch. As soon as I sat down, Jack told me that about a week earlier, Dr. Stone came toward him and threatened him with a raised fist, as if he were to punch him in the face. Jack was a short, middle-aged man with a paunch, and I could well imagine Dr. Stone, more than a head taller, coming at him with a raised arm. I only said:

"This is bad! I wouldn't expect this kind of behavior from a member of the medical staff!" Jack looked at me and slowly said:

"You know something? This Stone is an extremely nasty guy! I am sure that he hates me, not so much because of his trouble with privileges, but because, I think, he is an antisemite! I can feel it!"

Jack and I have been good friends for several years, and so I could allow myself to burst out laughing.

"What is it? What's funny?"

"Jack, listen! Stone is Jewish! I didn't know it until recently, when he accused you of being an antisemite! Isn't that funny?"

"He thought that I…? Well, I'll be…" and he too began to laugh.

"Jack, wouldn't it be better to stop this thing before Stone starts suing…?"

"Yeah… I'll talk to the urologists."

Then we both remembered that there was yet another doctor on our staff, a neurologist, Scott Sherman, also a tall, blond, Nordic looking guy, except that he had a big hook nose, which served better than an ID card. He was Jewish, and with that name, we wondered if he was born in the South...

Apropos the people who change their family name, I then told Jack of an episode that happened way back in the seventies when I lived in a suburb very close to NYC. We lived in a house near the coast and became quite friendly with our neighbors across the street. Their children played together with ours, we visited with each other, and sometimes we went together on weekend outings. One day this neighbor, Joe Schultze, came over and told me that he was going with his family for three weeks to Europe, and he would need a big favor. He asked cautiously:

"Peter, would it be OK, if I left your phone number at my office, in case they needed to contact me?"

"Of course, you may give our number. We'll gladly take a message for you."

"Thanks, but... I must tell you: they'll be asking for Wilson."

"What Wilson?"

"At work, they know me as Wilson! You know, how it is! Schultze is a foreign name; my ancestors came from Germany. In my business, it is best to have a good American name, like Wilson."

His business was to go to the radio and TV stations and arrange for airing advertisements for various products.

"You mean, with a German name, people might think that you were Jewish, and it might not be so good for business?"

"Oh, come on! It's not all that bad for the Jews!"

"A few months ago, you told me that you just joined the local Yacht Club!"

"What does that have to do —"

But I interrupted him:

"Did you join the club as Schultze, or as Wilson?"

"Wilson."

"Well, right after you told me about it, I also tried to join. They sent me a very polite letter, saying that the membership was full, up to capacity, and there was a very long waiting list…"

"Oh, I am sorry! That's not right! I didn't know they were like that!"

"That's what I mean: as Schulze, you might not have fared so well…" And we both remained silent for a few seconds. Then he continued:

"Peter, please, don't forget to tell Miriam! If they call from my office, they'll be asking for Wilson."

"Sure! Wilson! I'll tell Miriam."

"Thanks. I'll be contacting you from time to time to see if there was any message."

"No problem! Enjoy your vacation!" After Jack heard the story about my friend Schultze-Wilson, he made a troubled face and said:

"Yeah, my grandpa, too… changed our family name. He wanted a better life… free from experiences he had in Poland."

We finished our lunch, and before going back to work, Jack promised that he would see to it, that Stone receives the privileges that were due to him. Soon after our conversation, I heard the good news: the bitter turf fight had ended. The urologists relented and granted Dr. Stone privileges.

It was interesting to see that within the next two years, two more urologists joined our medical staff, as if to prove that the local turf was large enough to support many more urologists. And indeed, all of them had plenty of work. *

Through my diagnostic work with cancer, I was associated with a large group of local oncologists who ran a large office in town and enjoyed an excellent reputation. They saved or kept alive many people who were stricken with all sorts of cancer. When my cousin was suddenly

---

*The above stories bring out the issue of many immigrants changing their family name. It is a sad fact that most people change their family name just to avoid discrimination that arises from all sorts of prejudices. There are several episodes in this narrative that touch on a widespread problem in human society: the prejudice against "others". Prejudice is not a normal condition; children are born completely free of any prejudice. They get infected and corrupted by the adults, and so it is an acquired mental affliction, an illness residing in the human mind. Prejudice is also totally democratic: it infects all human races, and it exists, perhaps in a variable degree, in every culture and in all societies. I consider it as one of the personality disorders, and thus far, there is no known chemical medication to cure it. Experience has shown that, while it is very difficult to eliminate prejudice, it is possible to contain it to some degree, and in some people, it may be cured by sound reasoning and education. Prejudice is based on a preconceived judgment that is not grounded on facts, but is based on ignorance, fictions, and blind beliefs, deliberately spread by other members of society.

Prejudice against "others" is an evil condition, often associated with hatred of "others" and racism. As it is well known, virulent racism has facilitated crimes against minorities, and it often leads to murder and genocide. If one investigates the history of the world in the last 100 years, or as well the most recent events in the news, the results of hatred and prejudice are evident all around us.

diagnosed with a malignant tumor of lymph glands, too large to be removed surgically, I referred her to our oncologists. She was 65 years old, and I was told that at such an advanced age, her malignancy had a poor prognosis. Nevertheless, our oncologists started her on a protocol of chemotherapy, and within a short time, the X-rays showed an excellent response. Her tumor had shrunk to less than half size. The chemo was continued, and within a few weeks my cousin felt quite well.

However, one day, she called me up and complained that her medical insurance was "maxed out". To continue her chemo injections, she would have to pay thousands of dollars out of pocket! That sounded strange, and when I checked on the cost of her specific therapy, it turned out to be not at all so expensive. Then I found that she was receiving her injections in the office of our oncologists, and at a markup of over 200 percent, probably to cover the cost of labor, office maintenance and incidentals. I advised my cousin to transfer her medical records to an oncology office in her neighborhood and finish the course of treatment at a normal price. It all worked out very well. When I noticed that my cousin started buying lots of new clothes, I knew that she was completely cured of cancer. I remain forever grateful to our competent oncologists for saving her life. She lived 27 more years and reached the age of 92.

Practicing medicine in the last decades of the twentieth century was unavoidably entwined with business, and as a director of the laboratory, I was not spared from seeing some of its greedy underbelly. In the very first month of my second directorship, the lab urgently needed a new automated blood cell counter. The local salesman quoted a price that was much higher than what the same machine cost only six months earlier at my previous job location.

When I questioned the sudden large difference in price, the salesman explained:

"That low price is possible only out there, in the boonies! In this area, here, the price must be higher! We are in an expensive suburban region!"

After a prolonged negotiation, the salesman ultimately wanted to make a sale, and he finally accepted the same price as "in the boonies". I would soon find out why the price in the current location was so high. A higher price brings a larger commission, and if the lab manager happens to be agreeable with the high price, the salesman would reciprocate with a nice gift.

At about the same time, the lab also needed a new chemistry analyzer, and one day, a salesman surprised me with the following complaint:

"Your lab manager is interested in our chemistry analyzer, and I could show it here, in a neighboring hospital, but she is demanding that we fly her to California, for a demonstration at our main plant."

"Well, that's your call!" was all I said.

And so, the salesman gave in! My brazen lab manager was flown to California and spent four days to evaluate the automated chemistry analyzer. She did not recommend acquiring it, and I was 8glad, because I knew, it was not a good machine. The reason that we needed a new analyzer was, that the one on current lease, chosen by the previous manager, was thoroughly inefficient.

During the years of being director of pathology, I hired several assistant pathologists, and I quickly learned that letters of recommendation describing a candidate as "outstanding", were not to be relied upon. I had to conclude that some of the highest praises and most valedictorian letters were written for candidates who needed to be gotten out of the way and unloaded on someone else.

The very last of my assistant pathologists was hired in circumstances, that are best described as "different". About a year before I retired as director of the department, my second assistant pathologist retired, and I had an opening to fill. Just as I started to look for a replacement, the hospital administrator called me for a meeting in his office. The meeting was very brief; the administrator informed me that a psychiatrist was recruited to the hospital staff and suggested that I fill the position of assistant pathologist by engaging the psychiatrist's wife, who recently completed her residency training in pathology. This couple of physicians, the administrator explained, were immigrants from Eastern Europe; both had completed their specialty training in the US, and both came with outstanding recommendations. Knowing very well, what the term "outstanding" could bring about, I only said, I hoped she was well trained. Upon that, the administrator gave me a folder containing the file with credentials of the pathologist. I called and talked to the few individuals who signed the letters of recommendation, and my verbal inquiry did not reveal any problem. I gave the new pathologist a cursory interview, and within a week, she joined my staff.

The hospital's quality assurance policy required that all newly hired pathologists have a probationary period of three months, during which the director of the department had to check, verify and co-sign every diagnostic report. Only after the verification was completed and found satisfactory, the Director would issue a letter to the Quality Assurance Committee, and the new pathologist would then receive full staff privileges and be able to provide diagnostic reports independently.

Already during the first two weeks of supervision, I recognized that my new member of the department was not nearly ready to independently sign out diagnostic reports. After a full three months of supervision, I was compelled to extend the probationary period for another three months. Ultimately, during the entire period of six months, I ended up checking out, correcting, and signing every one of her diagnoses, and thus, I effectively carried a double workload. When I reported to the hospital administrator that my new assistant failed to perform at a satisfactory level and should be terminated, he implored me to be more patient and extend the supervision "a little longer". The administrator claimed that at that moment, he could not risk losing her husband, the psychiatrist.

I extended the probationary period for another three months, which was beyond any plan of the quality assurance policy. After having spent an enormous amount of time on supervision, I decided to invest some time in an attempt to teach and tutor her. We used the double-headed microscope, and on many occasions, she began to show some improvement. There was hope that with instruction and patience, my young assistant might eventually be able to work on her own.

On some occasions, this new assistant unwittingly gave me some comical relief. Once I walked into the lab while she was preparing a tissue for rapid frozen section diagnosis. This is done with a precision instrument, a microtome inside of a small freezer. Upon entering the room, I found my assistant banging with a heavy steel hammer against the microtome, vigorously trying to dislodge the frozen tissue from its plate. I asked her to stop hammering and showed her how to lift the tissue with a warm knife. I also began to understand how the steel plate of our precision instrument acquired several peculiar deep gouges. Later, after the frozen section diagnosis was relayed to the surgeon, I asked her:

"How could you use a hammer on the microtome? You know, it's a high-precision instrument!" She promptly explained:

"I had to use the hammer! My hands are not strong enough!"

As I looked at her in disbelief, she added with a sweet, amiable tone, implying a certain familiarity:

"Oh, you know, my father often used to tell me that I was like a słon v porcelane."

That last phrase was in her native Polish, and she quickly explained:

"The 'słon' in our language means 'an elephant'!"

"I see! But we don't use the elephant. We say: 'bull in a china shop'."

"Aha!"

I could see that her father knew his daughter very well. Thanks to my administrator's need of a psychiatrist, I acquired an assistant giving me innocent levity.

Continuing to work with this assistant, I was repeatedly jolted by instances where we both looked through the double-headed microscope at the same section of tissue, and she would come up with a diagnosis that was completely out of reality. She would diagnose an "invasive cancer" while looking at an area of cell degeneration with an atrophic reaction. That would be followed by a few perfectly rational diagnoses, but a few days later, while we both looked at a case of cancer, she would shock me by declaring a diagnosis of "degenerative change".

Finally, one day, my assistant clarified all our "misunderstandings". We were sitting at the double-headed microscope, and after I described to her in full detail all the signs that lead to a diagnosis of cancer of prostate, she proceeded to explain to me, why the diagnosis was still not evident. She put it this way:

"I know all the facts about this cancer, and I can see every one of the little details you just described, but still, all of them just don't fit together! It doesn't add up! Can you understand?"

"Can I...? Yes, I understand!"

There could be no better explanation! It was all so plain: the dots were all there, but the order in which to connect them was still missing. It was then, that I knew that any further attempt to teach her was bound to fail, and I gave up. Nine months of supervision and fruitless teaching left me saddled with an assistant who could not be allowed to work independently.

The last little story provided by this assistant occurred one morning when she walked into my office with her face all drawn down:

"Yesterday, I had a really bad day! Something terrible happened to my husband!"

"I am sorry! Is he OK?"

"This morning, he is better. Yesterday, he had a very bad accident."

"An accident? What happened?"

"He was treating one of his patients, you know, he was just quietly talking to him. This patient was, as usual, very quiet and depressed, but suddenly, out of the blue, he got up, knocked down a chair and a little table, and started punching my husband in the face, and he hit him in the mouth and nose, and in the eye! My husband says, he saw absolutely no sign that the patient was getting vexed or angry. Luckily, two male nurses heard the commotion and came into the room and restrained the patient."

"Well, I am glad he was quickly rescued!"

"No, no! It was not quick enough! My poor husband came home with a blue eye and broken lip, and a bloody nose and blood all over his jacket and shirt..."

"I am sorry to hear that! I hope he makes a speedy recovery!"

"Thank you!"

About a week later, she came into my office, closed the door, and very confidentially told me that her husband initiated a lawsuit against the hospital, based on "lack of proper protection during patient treatment." I warned her that he would lose his job, but she said, he wanted to quit anyway. There was a large community of immigrants from their country living in the vicinity, and her husband had already picked up a lot of private patients. Several days later, the psychiatrist was dismissed from the hospital staff.

Meanwhile, I began to feel tired of the directorship. One nice evening at home, I asked myself, *What do I need all this for? Especially the management part, which I never really enjoyed.*

In a nearby town practiced a capable, young and ambitious pathologist, more than 20 years my junior, who just recently left an academic position and became Director of Pathology in a local hospital. I thought he might like to take on a bigger position, and I could then retire as director and stay on for a while to work as a senior pathologist and his assistant. That way, I could get rid of management headaches and do what I always liked best: the diagnostic work. I proposed to the hospital administration to approach the young man and engage him as director…

It worked out, and the new director soon spread his wings over both hospitals. The transition was smooth, and I got a contract to stay on for one year and practice only diagnostic pathology on a 50 percent part-time schedule, that allowed us to do some traveling. In the end, I stayed on for a year and a half, and it was a good way to ease out into retirement, slowly and with pleasure.

In retirement for the past 21 years, I continue to keep well informed about issues in pathology and medicine in general, although much of the time, I am happily engaged in other activities: studying the history of art, visiting art museums and reading books or traveling.

I spent ten wonderful years volunteering in a local historic house and garden, where I enjoyed serving as a guide and docent, and learned a few things about horticulture and orchards. Now, this retired pathologist also has the pleasure of spending time recording his memories, and sometimes, he finds that the day doesn't have enough hours.

Chapter 17

The Business and Medicine

Having retired from my last active job, my involvement in pathology was limited to volunteering. I became an adjunct professor in a medical school on the West Coast, helping to teach in the student labs where I found that the modern course of pathology was integrated with internal medicine. The interest of the students was overwhelmingly devoted to internal medicine, while the subject of pathology was left behind. For example, while learning to recognize pneumonia, the students wanted only to see the X-ray image with a dense shadow in the lung, and they did not care to know about the underlying pathologic presence of liquid and inflammatory cells in the lung. I gathered that the new style of teaching medical students was adjusted to the modern way of practicing medicine. Another novelty was that medical students were no longer required to learn and store most of the information in their cortex. In the current century it seemed more important to learn and know where to find the information and how to use a proper algorithm. In that new ambiance, I soon lost interest in teaching, and two years later I quit.

In my new environment on the West Coast, I had a chance to be involved at the receiving end of the medical establishment. I found a family physician, a few specialists, and a dentist. As a patient, I observed that in this century, when a doctor, or more commonly, a physician's assistant (today called "physician's associate"), or a "nurse practitioner" sees a patient, they spend more time looking at the computer screen and entering data on the keyboard, than observing the patient. More recently, as COVID hovered in our background, a

"FaceTime" or a "Zoom" visit with a nurse practitioner, or less commonly, with a physician, became the new standard. It allows up to 30 minutes per visit in that new medium. That is usually followed by a short email communication with a summary of the visit. It seems that this alternative way of online digital visits will remain even after COVID has been tamed.

It appears that akin to the well-known term "military/industrial complex," medicine (today's "Healthcare") has been incorporated into an enormous new entity that may be called the "Insurance/Managed Care Complex," with the physicians squeezed between those two behemoths. * Among many other things, my healthcare company uses a new "managed care" standard for regular patient visits, the "six-minute" standard. The employed physician is allotted all of six minutes for a patient visit! More time is allowed if it is the very first visit.

The essence of the medical profession has changed. It has been transformed into a business. When I started studying medicine, choosing a medical profession felt almost like a calling. In any case, it used to be a profession that would offer lots of satisfaction and would be well rewarded. Above all, the profession was practiced with goodwill and with a first and foremost goal to do good for the patient. Physicians would follow the ancient Hippocratic Oath. As decades went by, we have come into a new century, a time when most physicians are now employed just like any other workers. There is a

---

* "Insurance/Managed Care Complex" is a term of my own. I have not seen any previous quote or copy of it, and I believe that it is an appropriate term. I did see a paper in JAMA: "Complexity in the US Health Care System Is the Enemy of Access and Affordability," which seems very much in line with my observations regarding business and its intrusion into medical practice (jamahealthforum. 2023.4430).

new jargon in which the word "medicine" is no longer used. The new word is "healthcare," and it is followed by "managed care". The whole system is run and dictated by professional managers whose main goal is profit. Medicine is certainly no longer a calling; it is now just a job, like grooming animals or feeding livestock. In this new managed care system, not only technologists, nurses and other medical personnel, but physicians too, are being manipulated and ordered how to practice their profession. As a result, some physicians have joined the union. I used to think that the duties of the medical profession were not compatible with the rules of a union, but now, with the new management of physicians, my feelings about that issue have changed.

As director of a hospital department, I had a vantage point to observe some of the dynamics between the business and medicine. During the last four decades of the twentieth century, medicine itself has undergone enormous advances and profound changes in the mode of its practice. During the same time, the business aspect of medicine and government regulations have undergone an even greater transformation, especially in the insurance and pharmaceutical industries and medical equipment manufacturing. All these advances brought with them a significant rise in cost. The erstwhile independent physicians have been first squeezed into group practices, and eventually into individual employment by large hospitals and clinics.

In the last two decades of the twentieth century, there have been great changes in how the medical insurance industry reimbursed hospitals, clinics and physicians. The insurance industry created a new order of hospital reimbursement: those hospitals that were able to quickly switch from in-patient care to the less costly out-patient care, would remain fiscally sound. The hospitals that did not make a quick transition to outpatient care, were falling into debt and were closed.

The hospitals had to find a new way to get out of financial difficulty. In the eighties, there was a time when swarms of consultants descended upon the hospitals to help them with financial management. That included a decrease in patients' length of stay (LOS) and advice in 'creative billing'. Later, in the nineties, there appeared a group of 'turn-around specialists' fiscal experts who knew how to turn around a hospital that was sinking in red ink and put it back on a more viable fiscal course. How did they do it? Their solution was to build either a whole new hospital or, more often, just an additional new wing, including a more modern operating suite with up-to-date X-ray equipment and a new emergency room. The 'turn-around specialist' became a part of the hospital management, usually acting as a highly paid CEO. His expertise was mainly in knowing how to obtain the funding for new construction. Before the construction even began, those funds, and often still only prospective funds or promissory notes, would effectively inject a new life into a moribund hospital.

The turn-around-specialists' skills were based on his connections with the financial world and with politicians, both on the state and federal levels. By means of convoluted channels and schemes, those connections were able to secure government guarantees for bonds floated by the hospital. Of course, the hospital owner would be eventually encumbered by a considerable debt obligation, but that would be payable over a long term, sometime in the future, in another era. While the new construction was only in the planning stages, the credit for the prospective bond funds would be liberally used as bait to extend the time for payments of current hospital debits and to get additional promissory notes. The bond machine had to be oiled, the obligations could wait till much later, and by the time the building blueprints were approved, and the construction work was ready to start, only a fraction of the original funding was still available to cover the actual cost of construction. If this sounds nebulous, vague, and complicated, it is indeed so, because it was much foggier and more convoluted than anyone could describe in a few lines. And yet, it was all done nicely, within the law.

Shortly after the construction was completed, there would be a big opening ceremony for the new building, with much praise for the CEO and all other deserving participants around him. In the first year after a new building was opened, the public would eagerly flock to the newest and most modern facility in town, and the hospital would for the first time in years show an annual profit. Then, within about a year, the 'turn-around expert' would quietly depart and move on to his next project, and the hospital would have to begin paying off the bond obligations.

This entire process of securing the guarantees for the bonds, obtaining the funds, finding a builder through a bidding process, preparing and approving the blueprints, and doing the actual construction would take approximately ten years. Working inside an institution, I was a witness to at least one such cycle, but I heard of and read about quite a few other such achievements, where a hospital was "turned around and put on a sound financial ground." The pattern was very similar; the final outcome would be seen by another generation and in another time.

As for the reimbursement of physicians (now called "the providers"), the insurance industry created a slew of obstacles, all aimed at withholding, delaying and denying payments for medical services, thereby increasing the profit of the insurance company. As the hospitals were forced to shift their activities from in-patient to out-patient care, the physicians who were previously dependent on a hospital salary were then encouraged to bill for out-patient services by themselves, although, by an agreement, a hefty part of those charges had to be turned over to the hospital.

The medical insurance industry created its own rules for billing, as did Medicare and Medicaid, by using a variety of different regulations, most requiring that the billing be done with the insurer's designated software. Medicare and Medicaid arbitrarily imposed a "cap," that is, a maximum payment for each physician's service or procedure. Such "capped" or "maximum" reimbursement fee amounted to about twenty percent of the "standard and usual fee" paid by the private insurance or by a private patient. It is this rule that caused (and still causes) some of the best, most qualified physicians to refuse to serve patients covered by Medicare and Medicaid. Even if a patient purchases secondary insurance to cover the difference between the Medicare-mandated payment and the "usual and standard" doctor's fee ("Medicare gap"), the total payment is still capped to the maximum allowed by Medicare or Medicaid! *

Additionally, if the clerical staff in a physician's office made an error and unknowingly charged a full fee for service to a Medicare-covered patient, such billing was taken as an infraction, punishable by law, and the physician would receive a threatening letter listing fines and other consequences of breaking the law. The various insurance companies also imposed their own schedules of payment for each medical procedure, set according to the contract with each employer (clinic or hospital). By means of having a separate contract with each clinic or hospital, the insurance companies were paying different fees for the very same procedure or service.

---

* Medicare and Medicaid were signed into a law in July of 1965, and then it took a bit of time before it was implemented.

As a hospital-based physician, I had the displeasure of participating in that system, and as an example, I still remember that for a PAP smear diagnosis, I was allowed to bill a Medicare patient no more than one dollar and fifty cents, which would hardly cover the expense of a stamp, paper and envelope, not to count the cost of informatics or the labor. For comparison, the "usual and standard fee" charged to a private patient for the same PAP smear was in the nineties about 7 to 8 dollars. Every now and then, I would receive from Medicare a "correction" on a previous payment, that is, a check amounting to one or two cents, certainly not worth the paper and envelope it was mailed with. One of those one cent checks I framed in my home office. And every few weeks, when my billing clerk sent an invoice with a standard fee for service, unaware that a young patient was for some unknown reason covered had Medicare, I would receive a letter from Medicare, threatening jail and fines if the invoice was not immediately corrected…

The medical insurance companies devised their own ploys to decrease or avoid payments of physicians' bills. The clerks of the insurance company were instructed to screen every submitted invoice and look for any smallest omission in patient data entry, and to use it as a pretext to ignore the entire bill. By the time the physician's office caught on to a missing payment, and by the time it was brought to the attention of the insurance company, the insurer's office would point out its own rule for "timely" billing, stating that "too much time had elapsed since the original date of service," and therefore, the outstanding bill was "no longer payable". As a result of this practice, the physicians would simply lose many payments for their services. At that time, I was lucky to have a most capable and diligent computer analyst who did all my billing and collected payments on 80 percent of my private bills. That high percentage of collection was quite unusual. From talking to my colleagues, I heard that most of their offices collected barely 50 percent of the payments due. The rest of their billing was written off. Of course, losing a Medicare or Medicaid payment was not a big loss, and one could consider it as going to 'goodwill'.

After decades of practice, and after years of having directed several labs, there is still one specific issue about the medical laboratories that presents for me a conundrum, a puzzle that I have never been able to understand. The law requires that for medical testing, all laboratories must purchase only FDA-approved equipment. Why, then, does the FDA still allow any medical lab to perform patient testing on its own "in-house" developed equipment and methodology without requiring FDA approval? Why does FDA not evaluate and approve all new proprietary equipment and methodology, before it is used on patients??

A case in point has been in the news over the past ten years in California, where the owner of a free-standing medical laboratory invented and patented her own equipment and methods of testing, and the lab was permitted to perform tests on thousands of patients and issue tens of thousands of medical test results, many of which had to be retracted because they were false. That lab has been closed, and its owners and principals were subject to court proceedings.

Perhaps one should not be surprised to see such freedom of enterprise in the field of medical laboratories, since we live in a system where millions of pills and other remedies are allowed to be sold "over the counter" without being checked and regulated for their content, to rule out any toxic substance, or to prove their effectiveness. These goods, most of them imported, are sold at the peril of those who buy them. It is: "laissez faire" and "caveat emptor". It is just like when you buy a bottle of wine or a piece of furniture: 'anything goes' and 'watch out for yourself'. Perhaps one should not be concerned, because, looking all around, the FDA has been doing a lot of good. It approved the vaccines and rapid tests for COVID in a record time.

At least some of the problems regarding products sold over the counter have been exposed in the press, for example, the high levels of toxic metals present in top brands of baby food (WSJ, Feb. 5, 2021) and hemp gummies, that send children into hospitals (WSJ Dec. 19, 2023). Assuming that these press reports are correct, shouldn't the content of food, at least for the babies and children, be checked and approved before being sold for consumption?

Chapter 18

Some Trends in Pathology

Concerning my professional work, practicing diagnostic pathology for over forty years, from the sixties to 2003, I felt a constant pressure from trend blazers in the CAP (College of American Pathologists) to adopt a slow, steady drift in making the cancer diagnosis, leading towards an "early diagnosis". This drift was not so much caused by new discoveries in the field of cancer. It was advocated after a simple recognition that if the diagnosis of cancer was made early, while the tumor was still small and did not spread too far, the prospect of eradicating cancer and completely curing the patient was close to a hundred percent. Consequently, the pathology leaders kept finding new ways to diagnose cancer in an ever earlier phase of its evolution. That was good, and it made sense, because early detection of cancer would certainly provide a better chance for a complete cure. However, as this trend has been pushed insidiously over many years, it was finally driven so far, that beyond a certain point, I was no longer able to follow it in my practice.

The pathologists at their annual meetings were offered a stream of new courses, many of them teaching how to make the diagnosis of cancer very, very early in its evolution. I attended those courses, and as far as I could see from an objective standpoint, some vague and inconstant observations in cell spread and appearance were declared sufficient to make a diagnosis of an "early cancer" and, thus, to alter the old, secure and established criteria for diagnosis. In this way, a diagnosis of cancer, I mean, real "invasive cancer," could be declared just a little sooner than it was there. Specific courses were advertised, with such titles as "How to Make an Early Diagnosis of Melanoma," or "Early Diagnosis of Breast Cancer," or "Carcinoma in situ" (= non-invasive!) in various organs. Simply put, the "early diagnosis" of cancer, whether in the breast, prostate, lung, colon, bone marrow, skin, or lymph glands, etc. became a dominant trend in pathology.

The result of this fad was that statistically, there appeared to be a rise in cancer incidence. Naturally, based on the presence of so many 'early discovered' cancers, many more people appeared to have a complete cure, a 'perfect outcome'. Simply put, in some cases this trend led to what I felt was an 'over-diagnosis' of cancer. I did not like it, and I avoided it in my practice. Over-diagnosis of cancer brings to the patient not only the stigma of having a malignancy, but also a personal anguish, and down the road, the difficulty in obtaining a job or life and medical insurance.

Two events in the seventies that closely coincided in time, made the new trend towards over-diagnosis of cancer only stronger. At the time, two brave ladies, the spouse of the President and the spouse of the Vice-President of the US, publicly announced that they had cancer of the breast. With such news, everyone became aware of breast cancer, and an unprecedented number of women started to have check-ups and mammography, and all of this was very good and positive. What we saw next was a great increase in the incidence of breast cancer, but much of it was only 'in situ' (non-invasive) and not at all the real, invasive cancer.

At the time, the treatment for invasive breast cancer was radical surgery with the removal of the breast and a part of the chest muscles and all axillary lymph glands. The removal of all lymph glands in the armpit caused swelling and considerable disability of the arm below. Moreover, an aggressive surgeon at a well-known hospital even advocated doing a "sample biopsy" of the opposite breast, just as a precaution. An entire "simple mastectomy" would be done just for a "carcinoma in situ", a borderline tumor that might never advance to become a true invasive cancer.

Not only was it an era of aggressive cancer diagnosis, but it was also a time of over-aggressive surgery. It took more than a decade before a less radical approach to breast cancer was applied by doing a removal of only the lump of tumor with a thin layer of surrounding tissue, a "lumpectomy," with only a sampling of two or three sentinel lymph glands. This was a much less extensive surgery, which was not so debilitating, but yielded results that were equally good as the radical surgery. In the interim, too many women were subjected to a simple mastectomy without having any evidence of true, invasive cancer, and too many had radical surgery with the removal of all local lymph glands and part of chest muscles. Most women who underwent a mastectomy for "in-situ cancer" would not have chosen that procedure if they had been aware that they could live safely, having removed only the tumor lump, and continuing with regular clinical check-ups.

The tumors of the skin are another area, where many people have been over-diagnosed as having either a "malignant melanoma" or an "early squamous cell carcinoma". That problem was compounded when dermatologists decided to include the pathology of skin into their own specialty. They created for themselves a short training program leading to a certificate in dermatologic pathology, and effectively took over the field of skin pathology. Thus, a dermatologist would take a biopsy of the skin, and a dermatologist would make a diagnosis. The only problem was that the dermatologists received training that was limited only to skin pathology, without having to learn the pathology of the entire body. Such narrow, one-sided training made it hard to make a diagnosis of the less common variants of skin tumors or of such complex and multifaceted tumors as malignant melanomas.

In the sixties, there was a textbook of skin pathology, "Histopathology of the Skin", written by a dermatologist, Walter Lever, MD, who was trained in Germany. I first saw that textbook when I was a resident in pathology training, and I still remember the chapter on the nevus versus malignant melanoma. That textbook (sixties edition) espoused a special philosophy in making a diagnosis of malignancy. It advised that if "atypical cells" were present within a nevus, it was best to call it a malignant melanoma because "atypical cells would anyway become a melanoma"! After reading that reckless opinion, I never used that textbook again. I believed, as my teachers had taught me, that one should never call anything malignant - before it is proven to be malignant. Through the decades of practicing pathology, I had seen too many cases of "malignant melanoma" or "early squamous cell carcinoma" of skin that were, upon review correctly diagnosed as "atypical nevus" or "actinic keratosis," and saved the patient from unnecessary radical surgery or other therapy for a malignancy. The problem was compounded by the fact that human skin is covered by multiple nevi, and very often, one may find a nevus with a few atypical cells, which is still not a malignant melanoma.

Another very different example of over-diagnosis of cancer of the skin is the so-called "basal cell carcinoma", which, despite its name, is not a true, invasive cancer. This tumor, known as the "most frequent type of cancer of skin," is generally a benign tumor. The name "basal cell carcinoma" was given back in 1902 by Dr. Edmund Krompecher, and the name stuck. Although its growth shows local invasion of the skin, by general rule, it does not develop distant metastases, and therefore, by definition, it is not a true cancer. It presents either as a skin nodule or as a chronic ulcer that does not heal. It is mostly caused by sun radiation (UV), and it usually appears on the parts of the skin most exposed to sunlight. This tumor is also known under a more appropriate name: "ulcus rodens" (=persistent ulcer) or "basal cell epithelioma" (basal cell epithelial tumor), names that correctly denote its benign nature. As with all non-invasive, benign tumors, a simple complete excision presents a cure.

It has also been shown that the diagnosis of "early prostate cancer" does not require immediate therapy. Many prostate cancer patients who were in the last 30 years subjected to surgery or radiation or chemotherapy, will nowadays, if given a choice, prefer to be monitored by observation and thus spare themselves from deleterious side-effects of surgery or radiation. By choosing observation and checkups, those patients enjoy a better quality of life. It has been shown that most of the "low grade" cancers of the prostate do not grow aggressively, and most people diagnosed with that type of 'cancer' have a normal life span without any radical treatment.

As I continue to follow the professional literature concerning diagnostic pathology, I notice with great satisfaction that recently, the general trend has been swinging back towards a more normal, balanced, objective diagnosis of cancer. In the last few years, the trend of over-diagnosis of cancer, disguised as an 'early cancer diagnosis', is finally being recognized as exaggerated and it is slowly being reversed. Occasional reports about this reversal may be seen in medical literature and even in the daily press. Here is a reference to the article: "Over-diagnosis of Noninvasive Tumors Following Organized Breast Cancer Screening", by Kelly Young, published in Medical News/Physician's First Watch, Jan.10, 2017, with the original article by Karsten J. Jørgensen, MD et al. in Annals of Internal Medicine, 2017. This paper shows that in a large study of breast cancer patients, one out of three patients was treated unnecessarily; they had no cancer.

In line with this good new trend, it has been recently proposed that some "early forms of in-situ cancer" should be called only descriptively, just what they are: "atypical cells" (not cancer!), signaling that there was no need for aggressive surgical therapy and that monitoring by regular check-ups would suffice.

I always remember the principles taught while I was still in training: 'atypical cells' should not be called cancer, unless one can see definite criteria for that diagnosis. And those straightforward criteria for diagnosis of invasive cancer require two major findings: that the growth unequivocally invades the adjacent tissue by highly atypical, true cancer cells and that it is recognized as capable of producing a distant metastasis. Without those characteristics, a tumor should not be called cancer. All those growths called "in situ" (= in place) are not true cancers. Calling cancer too early is harmful to the patient. There is a general principle in medicine that was known to Romans 2,000 years ago: "Primum non nocere!" (= First, do no harm!). In our modern time, this old principle seems to have been forgotten.

There is a recent trend among professional leaders and educators in pathology to teach the current pathologists how to avoid over-diagnosis of cancer. The proof of this new development can be found in the list of current courses for pathologists. These modern courses teach that an accurate diagnosis of cancer is more important than a too early diagnosis. Here are some examples:

> 1. "Masqueraders of Malignancy in Breast Pathology: Strategies and Solutions" the title speaks for itself. There have been too many unwarranted diagnoses of cancer in cases that only masquerade or 'look like' cancer, and it describes a method to avoid it.
>
> 2. "Benign Mimics of Myelodysplastic Syndromes and Myeloproliferative Neoplasms: How to Avoid the Common Pitfalls." Here, one learns about the benign mimickers of malignancy in blood cancer (leukemia).

3.   "Common Errors in Diagnosing Chronic Colitis and the Challenges of Inflammatory Bowel Disease-associated Dysplasia." another area where "dysplasia" should not be mistaken for cancer of colon. The description of the 'challenges' underscores the importance of understanding the pathways and stages leading from inflammatory/reactive states to benign tumors, and later, but only potentially, to a malignancy.

4.   "Spectrum of Colitis, Dysplasia, and Cancer in inflammatory Bowel disease." Here again, "dysplasia" means 'atypical cells' or a change that may sometimes lead to cancer but usually remains unchanged.

In summary, there has been quite a turn-around in the criteria required for cancer diagnosis, a great improvement over what was happening in the previous five decades. The trend of over-diagnosis is out, and the current course in pathology is to make the diagnosis as accurate as possible. One might ask, why did so many errors in pathologic diagnosis represent an over-diagnosis of malignancy? The answer is that some physicians choose to practice defensively, which is an easy way to avoid missing a diagnosis of cancer. But the "easy way" may not be a good way!

An enormous improvement in diagnostic pathology within the last thirty years involves the increasing use of modern diagnostic methods: immune histochemical staining of tissues, with or without enzyme digestion, application of genetics, molecular PCR, etc. These methods are nowadays done using highly automated equipment. Thus, a scientific technique in methodology has largely replaced the 'art' of the pathologist, who was making the diagnosis of cancer subjectively, by simple observation through a microscope. In short, the medical art in pathology is being replaced by science-based technology.

The clinical accuracy of science-based testing for cancer, performed on automated, computer-driven equipment is superior, so long as the quality controls fall within two standard deviations, which will guarantee an accuracy of 98 percent or better. Very little in the realm of biology is "one hundred percent", because outliers and exceptions abound. With 98 percent accuracy, the automated machines make fewer mistakes than an average pathologist with a microscope. What will then happen to the role of the pathologist in modern medicine? That role is rapidly diminishing, and recent statistics already show that the number of practicing pathologists has been significantly reduced.

Did the electron microscope ever become the ultimate tool for making a pathologic diagnosis? In the fifties and sixties, practically any published images of biological material taken with the high power of an electron microscope represented a new discovery that could be published as "basic research". In the seventies and early eighties, the pathologists' meetings regularly offered a major course in electron microscopy. The course was given with the implication that electron microscopy would in the future play a big role in making accurate pathological diagnoses. That future never materialized!

Meanwhile, new methods based on immune chemical staining showed a more promising role, and pathologists were offered new courses in this methodology, while the electron microscopy was set aside. I attended one course on immune staining methods, where the lecturer started his talk by showing the image of an electron microscope, with a large "FOR SALE" sign hanging on it. The implication was quite clear. The electron microscope has remained mainly a research tool. Its role in diagnostic pathology is minimal, reduced to only a couple of diseases of kidneys in a very early stage. Immune histochemistry and other modern methods have taken over.

In the clinical testing laboratories, the pathologists have been largely replaced by technologists or by doctoral scientists (PhDs). The role of the diagnostic surgical pathologist has been reduced to a small spectrum of simple diagnoses of hernia, inflammation, degenerative changes, benign tumors, infections, review of 'positive' cytologic samples, and simple diagnosis of cancer, usually without a precise definition of subtype. However, efficient cancer therapy can be achieved only by specially designed protocols for each cancer subtype.

Pathology, like all the rest of medicine, has become more science-based and less of an 'art'. In general, the art component in medicine now plays an ever-diminishing role. Some people go as far as hoping that artificial intelligence (AI) and computerized equipment with algorithms might largely replace the physicians. For now, that remains a doubtful and dangerous proposition…

During the years of practicing pathology, I was occasionally asked a challenging question:

"Will the doctors ever find a way to eradicate cancer?"

This question always reminded me of President Nixon's "war on cancer", where he issued 100,000-dollar grants to individual physicians/researchers, chosen without much regard for the quality of their achievements. To answer the question of whether cancer can ever be eliminated, one first needs to remember that cancer is a biological phenomenon, a part of the Nature, and that Nature provides constant changes. Way back, 2,500 years ago, ancient Greeks knew that the only constant thing in Nature was the change itself. As they said in Greek: "panta rhei" (= everything flows). The Nature, that is, all living organisms, flora and fauna, are always changing and are endowed with the ever-present phenomenon of mutation and evolution. Mutation creates a "moving target", which constantly evolves and transforms itself. As we learn to cure one type of cancer, a new variant appears, just like currently the newer variants of Covid virus. In addition to mutation, there is an ever-increasing pollution of air, water, soil, and food. All these factors contribute to more cancer, and when it comes to the question of ever eliminating cancer, unfortunately, my answer is negative.

A further reason for failing to fully eradicate cancer is that the cause of cancer is not one, but many. There are numerous factors causing cancer; some are chemical, like nicotine and asbestos; some are viral (HIV, EBV) or it is radiation, and less commonly, various known and unknown genetic defects. Finally, there are causes of cancer, which are, as of now, entirely unknown. To complicate the origin of cancer, some people possess immune and other defense factors that protect them from cancer. For example, why is it that there are millions of heavy smokers who never get cancer of lung? Moreover, there are some very heavy smokers who live to be over 90 years old and die of natural causes! This also explains how the tobacco industry was able to "prove" for decades that cigarettes did not cause cancer. That deception was helped by 'scientists/researchers', who were well paid and willing to publish papers and even a whole book claiming that tobacco was harmless. People believed it, and some still believe it, like those who want to believe that COVID is "just like any flu".

Cancer is a multifactorial disease, meaning that it has more than one factor causing it. Human defense against cancer is also multifactorial. Every individual has more than one factor of defense against cancer. Some of these factors are possibly of immune type or are embedded in the genes. We still do not know all those factors, and without that knowledge, how could we possibly devise a cure that will eradicate all different cancers? Thus, I must come out with a pessimistic answer that at this time we are not even close to being able to eradicate cancer, and it may be realistic only to hope that in the next few decades, at least some specific types of cancer will become curable. *

Current research conducted in genetics offers a glimmer of hope by the prospect of a new therapy that would cure cancer or other diseases by changing or eliminating a single faulty gene. It has been shown that some rare types of cancer are caused by a single mutation of a gene, and those cancer types might be thus cured. The future of genetic treatment of cancer and other diseases looks very bright, but research towards gene therapy opens serious concerns with ethical issues. Altering the human genome may have unforeseen consequences...

---

* When thinking of multiple immune and other factors protecting us from cancer or infections, factors which have not been detected and remain unknown, it is pertinent to remember the fact that about one half of HIV-infected people have been reported as remaining free of AIDS disease ten years after becoming HIV-positive. This means that about one half of all HIV-positive persons carry some natural factors which protect them from getting ill with AIDS.

In the early days of HIV testing, after 1985, for every one person who was sick with AIDS, there were about seven other people who were HIV-positive but not at all sick.

Also, with COVID, there are many cases, where a couple living together reports one as having been ill with COVID, while the other stayed completely free of illness, though both tested positive for COVID. There is a lot more around immunity that has yet to be discovered.

Conclusion

Some of the above assembled stories may give the impression that a large part of my professional life was a hard, constant fight, full of negative experiences. This is not the case. The episodes and stories gleaned from my memories occupy a relatively small segment of time, out of more than forty years of active practice. In fact, this entire narrative describes only a small fraction of time out of all those long years. Overall, most of the time, my professional work was filled with satisfaction, and there were numerous occasions when my job gave me real pleasure. To make an important, valid, correct diagnosis, especially in a very difficult case, or to solve a case that "did not read the book", gave me each time a big thrill. There were countless times when I was happy over one or another good event or favorable patient outcome. In the forty-odd years, there was a legion of examples where my job gave me true fulfillment, and here follow a few brief examples that have stayed forever fresh in my memory.

Early on in my academic practice, a patient was admitted to the hospital for treatment of a sarcoma (connective tissue cancer) of the lower leg. He was scheduled to have an amputation of his leg. As is customary, I reviewed the microscopic slides of his tumor biopsy from another hospital and found that it was a rare tumor of sweat gland origin, and it was benign, an adenoma. After my diagnosis was confirmed by expert consultation, the amputation was canceled, and the patient was discharged from the hospital and went happily home.

Then there was a case where a patient was supposed to have extensive plastic surgery on her face for an "early skin cancer." When I reviewed her original microscopic slides from another hospital, I found only actinic keratosis, a benign, possibly "precancerous" skin condition, caused by excessive sun exposure. The diagnosis was confirmed by an expert consultation, and the patient was saved from unnecessary surgery.

I encountered in my practice a number of patients referred to the hospital with a diagnosis of malignant melanoma of skin, but upon review, they had only an atypical nevus, which did not require any therapy at all. I have also seen quite a few patients who were originally diagnosed with a malignant lymphoma (lymph gland tumor), and who, upon review of the original biopsy had only lymphoid hyperplasia (a benign overgrowth of lymphoid cells) and needed no further treatment.

Similar fortunate occurrences continued throughout my practice, and they always brought me pleasure and satisfaction.

Most physicians I worked with were compassionate, ethical, devoted and diligent individuals, doing good for their patients. The few "bad apples" that I did run across, represented only aberrations, such as may be found within any profession and in all corners of humanity.

During 25 years as director of a department, I was fortunate to work with two assistant pathologists of excellent quality, both on a personal and on a professional level. Each one of them stayed with me for eleven years, and each provided unmatched assistance. Dr. Usha Kavuri, who I hired out of training for her very first job as an attending pathologist, was smart, diligent, responsible and of the highest integrity. Dr. Adam Pumaren was no less sharp, able, competent, devoted to his work, highly ethical, and prudent. Both were not only my long-standing co-workers, but above all, they had become my friends.

By the nature of my profession, many of my memories dwell on cancer. I want to remind the reader that when one surveys the entire enormous variety of tumors in humans, the outlook is not so gloomy.

The statistics clearly show that most of tumors are benign and relatively harmless. A cancer diagnosis is important and requires far more attention, but fortunately, cancer represents only a relatively small minority of tumors in humans.

I want to point out that, as it is in life, the events that are casual, normal, and "usual", are simply taken for granted, and will thus be of a lesser interest. Therefore, when it comes to choosing a subject for a story, the good or banal or natural events will be mostly left out. Life is like a field of clover: one does not pay attention to the thousands of plants with three leaves, but the eye searches for the less common, the rare or unusual, the clover with four leaves. It is those events that appear odd, rare, unexpected, out of the ordinary, weird, bad, surprising, aberrant, or in any way 'abnormal' that always evoke a greater interest, and it is only for this reason, that many episodes in this narrative describe subjects or occurrences that were curious, uncommon, adverse, or anomalous. After all, let us remember that my profession and my specialty is called pathology, which is defined as the science about the sick, the abnormal. And when it comes to the live organisms as complex as the humans, one will always easily find plenty of sickness and pathology, issues and appearances that are outside of the ordinary or normal, either in physical or mental sense. And to make it more difficult, the Nature has provided us with lots of conditions which dance right around the border of what is expected as 'normal'. There is no sharp line of division.

Some of this narrative involves personal experiences that were neither nice nor pleasant, but "such is life!" Not all of it smells like roses. While I speak of personal experiences, I want to emphasize that most of the people I came across in my career were upright, good, and decent individuals. Of course, I could not help recognizing that some people I got to know in my travels carried with them certain baggage that rendered them quite undesirable. Instances where one meets individuals exhibiting rude, egotistic, and heartless behavior may be encountered in every society. Most of such individuals are either not very bright or are plainly obtuse. Unfortunately, we also may encounter highly intelligent, smart people who use their power of thinking to advance wrong causes and to create ugly schemes or to misinform and take advantage of "others". Keeping a balance on the tightrope of dealing with such 'difficult' people requires great patience and endurance, some ingenuity, and a good measure of painful tolerance… One may ask whether most of the individuals inhabiting this Earth are fine, decent, righteous people possessing a moral conscience and caring about all others, or are most humans just selfish, greedy characters who care only for their personal benefit? Judging by the outcome of the 2024 election in the US, what should be the answer to the above question concerning our American society? Each one of us must conclude according to her or his conscience.

By choice, I spent my entire professional career in the North-East of US, and I was fortunate to work in an environment where majority of people were civil and reasonable, exhibiting good and tolerant behavior. I was happy to live and work in an ambiance where most folks were able to see that the Earth was not flat and I found that most of the people around me possessed the power of reasoning, strong enough to keep their minds free from baseless beliefs and prejudices. Overall, my years of work gave me pleasure, and a large part of it came from being in company of good people.

A Personal Note

I am grateful to my parents for their decision to bring me into life and let me feel their love for the few years they were able to be with me.

I am grateful to the good and brave people who saved my life and provided for me when my parents were taken away and destroyed.

I thank all my ancestors for the genes they passed on to me.

I thank the Nature for having assembled those genes into a mosaic that formed a person able to lead a balanced and productive life.

Above all, my gratitude goes to my dear wife, my friend, companion and the love of my life, for choosing me to mix her genes with and make us a beautiful family.

Special thanks go to my oldest daughter who read this manuscript in its early unedited form. and gave many invaluable suggestions and comments.

This record is made primarily for my family and friends. Within two or three generations, it will be lost and forgotten. But I am leaving behind something that will remain for a much longer time: the genes carried forward by my progeny for as long as Nature will allow. Those genes will show up again, arranged in new mosaics that will carry parts of my spirit and will continue to follow the laws of Nature.

www.ingramcontent.com/pod-product-compliance
Lightning Source LLC
Chambersburg PA
CBHW051535020426
42333CB00016B/1946